Dr. Pascarelli's Complete Guide to Repetitive Strain Injury

Dr. Pascarelli's Complete Guide to Repetitive Strain Injury

What You Need to Know about RSI and Carpal Tunnel Syndrome

Emil Pascarelli, M.D.

WILEY

John Wiley & Sons, Inc.

Copyright © 2004 by Emil Pascarelli. All rights reserved

Published by John Wiley & Sons, Inc., Hoboken, New Jersey
Published simultaneously in Canada

Design and production by Navta Associates, Inc.

Illustrations credits: pages 11, 12, 13, 14, 16 (top), 49, 61, 79, 152 (both), 154 (top and bottom), and 156 courtesy of Ahmet Sinav, M.D.; pages 16 (bottom) and 24 reprinted with permission from *Scientific American Medicine*; page 46 reprinted from B. M. Sucher. 1990. Thoracic outlet syndrome: A myofascial variant. Part I: Pathology and diagnosis. *The Journal of American Osteopathic Association* 90 (8): 471–479; pages 136 and 142 reprinted with permission from Flexrest.com; page 172 (top, both) reprinted with permission from the Smithsonian Institution; page 191 reprinted with permission from David Lloyd Rivinus.

The information contained in this book is not intended to serve as a replacement for professional medical advice. Any use of the information in this book is at the reader's discretion. The author and publisher specifically disclaim any and all liability arising directly or indirectly from the use or application of any information contained in this book. A health care professional should be consulted regarding your specific situation. The author has no financial connection to the manufacturers of the equipment or products mentioned in this book. These materials are considered to be of clinical interest in the treatment of repetitive strain injury (RSI).

For general information about our other products and services, please contact our Customer Care Department within the United States at (800) 762-2974, outside the United States at (317) 572-3993 or fax (317) 572-4002.

Wiley also publishes its books in a variety of electronic formats. Some content that appears in print may not be available in electronic books. For more information about Wiley products, visit our web site at www.wiley.com.

Library of Congress Cataloging-in-Publication Data:

Pascarelli, Emil F., date.
  Dr. Pascarelli's complete guide to repetitive strain injury : what you need to know about RSI and carpal tunnel syndrome / Emil Pascarelli.
    p. cm.
  Includes bibliographical references.
  ISBN 0-471-38843-2 (paper : alk. paper)
  1. Overuse injuries–Popular works. 2. Carpal tunnel syndrome–Popular works. I. Title.
  RD97.6.P368 2004
  617.1'72–dc22
                                                                        2004002610

To my wife, Dolores Klein Pascarelli, my daughter, Claudia Pascarelli Lyon, and my son, Eric Pascarelli, without whom this book could not have been created

It is the familiar that usually eludes us in life.
What is before our nose is what we see last.

–Sir William Barrett

Contents

Foreword

When Dr. Emil Pascarelli founded the Miller Health Care Institute for Performing Artists in 1985, he could hardly have appreciated the pioneering nature of his vision. Nor could he have realized the profound effect his novel and painstaking approach would have on the way physicians would come to view performance and workplace injuries. Under Pascarelli's direction, the Institute at Columbia University in New York became one of the largest clinics in the country treating repetitive strain injuries. Growing to about a thousand patients a month, with musicians, dancers, and keyboard workers of all varieties, an enormous experience was developing. Even after many previous fruitless consultations and treatments, patients benefited from the application of a meticulous medical and ergonomic approach, which was complemented by comprehensive upper body biomechanical assessment, laboratory tests, and finally routine videotaping of a patient's customary activity. An integrated program of ergonomic modification and a highly refined treatment program achieved success and rehabilitation even for the chronically afflicted.

Dr. Pascarelli recognized that the workplace had evolved from the backbreaking and lung-challenging labors of previous centuries to the unique demands of the modern office. Repetitive strain injury (RSI) now makes up more than 60 percent of work-related illnesses. Dr. Pascarelli recorded subtle differences in the manner in which workers performed their jobs, and how some become disabled. He recognized the significant physical demands on what he termed the "sit-down athlete," and how poor biomechanical work habits or poor ergonomic design can lead to injury-causing behaviors such as the disabling keyboard habits of "leaners, loungers, and clackers."

Unfortunately, outside of the institute, the approach to patients with "overuse" syndromes had evolved in a somewhat chaotic clinical environment, with each specialty focusing on one or another familiar characteristic. Often the diagnosis was based on the most prominent symptom rather than on the recognition that tendinitis or carpal tunnel syndrome may be part of a larger constellation of symptoms, the recognition of which would lead to the real etiology of a patient's disability. The poor diagnostic results derived from the unfortunate erosion of physicians' clinical skills, a reliance on limited physical examinations, and moving too quickly to highly focused laboratory tests. In this setting, equivocal or incomplete test results are often accorded undue significance, even in the face of contradictory physical findings. These misleading clues often divert one's attention—to the detriment of the patient and the frustration of the clinician when the expected "cure" doesn't materialize.

Returning to basics, Dr. Pascarelli, through his highly diligent approach, brought order out of chaos. He emphasized the fundamental characteristic common to all these injuries: a history of repetitive use of the upper extremities in an intense and often awkward fashion.

The lessons learned redefined the terms of cumulative trauma, repetitive strain injury, and overuse syndrome. His "Sherlock Holmes" approach, considering every clinical clue rather than discounting those that do not fit a preconceived diagnosis, has rescued many patients from the distressing labyrinth of multiple diagnoses, failed therapies, and increasingly frustrating consultations. This clinical approach was based on evidence that despite initial symptoms in the fingers, hands, and arms, work-related upper-extremity disorders constitute a diffuse neuromuscular illness characterized by significant upper-body disturbances that affect function in the arms, hands, and fingers. Once therapy is targeted at the proper neck and shoulder sites, the symptoms begin to disappear.

Now, in addition to the benefits to the many thousands of patients at the institute, Dr. Pascarelli has given us an invaluable resource, a welcome distillation of his unique experience, equally valuable to patients, their families, therapists, and physicians. This book guides the reader through an otherwise daunting maze in the company of a skilled and compassionate healer.

There is invaluable advice on managing pain, and a constructive approach to physical and occupational therapy. Careful analysis of thousands of videotapes of people working and musicians playing has led to accurate data on the ergonomics and biomechanics of upper extremity and neck and shoulder disorders. Rational decisions can now be made regarding workstation modifications as well as mitigating the rigors of daily living. This guidance is all the more valuable coming from a physician-investigator who has, perhaps more than any other specialist, "walked the walk." Physicians, therapists, and patients reading this book now have a unique opportunity to look over the shoulder of one of the foremost RSI specialists as he goes about his work.

It is always a major benefit to the health care community when an astute clinician-scientist critically evaluates an extensive and unusually successful practice, and then carefully documents the lessons learned. This readable book is a gift to us all: workers, patients, therapists, and physicians, as well as all who would ensure a safe and productive workplace.

Herbert I. Machleder, M.D.
Emeritus Professor of Surgery
University of California, Los Angeles

Preface

Each year we learn more about how to diagnose and manage repetitive strain injury (RSI), a disorder still poorly understood by many. With this book, I hope to clear up some of the mystery. My own experience has taught me that RSI is no more difficult to diagnose than many other medical illnesses. The confusion occurs because it is usually work-related, and caused by many factors. Yet a good history and complete physical examination by an interested physician can arrive at the diagnoses necessary for successful treatment.

Posture plays a key role in the genesis of this disorder. Poor posture can lead to nerve impairment and subsequent soft-tissue effects on the entire upper body. RSI is real—not a product of your imagination—and can become a chronic disability if left untreated. We have also become more sophisticated in the treatment of RSI as we observe people improving with focused physical therapy; home exercises; and ergonomic, biomechanical, psychological, and medical interventions. This book reflects my personal observations of patients as well as the research work of many others in the field. My hope is that better understanding of this illness will lead the way to recovery for the many persons afflicted with RSI.

Acknowledgments

Many people, both directly and by their influence, have contributed to making this book possible.

Thanks to Lisa Sattler, M.S., P.T., a talented and extraordinarily caring physical therapist and lecturer, for all her help and advice with the exercise program and other therapies grounded in her long experience with RSI patients. Vera Wills, professor of graduate pedagogy at the Manhattan School of Music, an insightful and skilled ergonomist and educator, made important contributions to chapters 8 and 12. To Yu-Pin Hsu, M.M., M.S., OTR/L, Ed.D., for wearing two hats: accurately notating my patient exams, which were so important for this book, and contributing elements of her doctoral research. Thanks to Ariel Stoll, who was extremely helpful in assisting me with my patients.

I would like to thank medical illustrator Ahmet Sinav, M.D., for his fine work in producing many of the illustrations. Dr. Herbert I. Machleder, emeritus professor of surgery at UCLA Medical School, kindly wrote the foreword of this book and in our many discussions on RSI spurred me on with his enthusiastic encouragement. Dr. Sidney J. Blair, emeritus professor of orthopedic surgery at Loyola University, was an important source of ideas and support. My longtime colleague Martin Cherniack, M.D., M.P.H., professor of medicine at the University of Connecticut Health Center and director of the Ergonomics Technology Center there, was a knowledgeable and inspired collaborator on patient care.

John J. Kella, Ph.D., was a valuable associate early in my work on RSI in musicians. I also would like to thank Professor Tom Armstrong, Ph.D., of the University of Michigan College of Engineering and director of the Center for Ergonomics there, and David Rempel, M.D., professor of medicine at the University of California, San Francisco, and director of the Ergonomics Program there, for the inspiration that their work on RSI provided me. The astute work of Stuart B. Leavitt, Ph.D., on eye problems was a valuable resource. I also would like to thank the editors of the *Journal of Occupational Rehabilitation* and Kluwer Academic/Plenum Publishers for allowing me to quote some of my research results. Bruce Hymanson, P.T., the inventor of Bodyblade, and his wife, Carrie Hymanson, P.T., offered skillful advice on upper-body treatment methods. Thanks to Perry Ritter for his talented ergonomic modifications of musical instruments, which made it possible for many injured musicians to continue their careers. Thanks to Hugh McLoone, ergonomist and usability researcher at Microsoft, for keeping me up to date on the latest technical innovations in computer equipment.

Thanks to Thomas W. Miller, executive editor, John Wiley & Sons, for his editorial support and patience in making this book possible and to Nicholas Bakalar for his skillful editing and organization of the manuscript. Harvey Klinger, my agent, was a staunch supporter and communicator of my efforts.

Introduction

Medicine, like law, should make a contribution to the
well-being of workers and see to it that, so far as possible,
they should exercise their callings without harm. So, I for
my part have done what I could and have not thought it
unbecoming to make my way into the lowliest workshops
and study the mysteries of the mechanical arts.

—Bernardino Ramazzini, 1713

You may have experienced discomfort or pain in your hands,
wrists, arms, shoulders, or neck. Perhaps you are only sensing
mild discomfort, but are beginning to fear something more serious. If you've noticed that these symptoms appear while you're
doing repetitive work or just after you've stopped doing it, if you
are in discomfort for your entire workday and beyond, you have
reason to be concerned. You may be facing repetitive strain
injury (RSI) in its early stages.

What you need is a guide to understanding RSI and what
you can do about it. Finding the right doctor, the right diagnosis,
and the right treatment requires understanding a complex problem that even most doctors are not trained to handle.

If your injury has persisted for some time, you may have been to one or more specialists. Opinions can differ from specialist to specialist depending on their experience with RSI. You may have been given medications, wrist splints, neck braces, and exercises, but if nothing you've tried has had more than a temporary effect on your pain or other symptoms, you need this book.

Many of my patients complain that health professionals, employers, and often fellow employees don't understand what they are going through. Because RSI has no obvious visible signs, the implication is that it is all in your mind, you're a hypochondriac, a slacker, a malingerer. You simply don't want to get better. Worldwide, people are finding that they have to defend themselves against these charges, sometimes explicit and at other times implied, when all they want is to get better and be themselves again.

A study of fifty-two Australian women with RSI whose work ranged from typing to poultry processing shows that the problem is universal and far from resolved. These women were interviewed about their search for help from physicians and health care providers. The study, which was aptly called "Pilgrimage of Pain," quotes one of the women interviewed:

> and then people tell you there can't be anything wrong with you. I said, "Look, I've had five children. I know pain. I know how it feels. I know when it's gone and I do feel pain. Don't tell me I don't feel pain because I know pain. I'm not stupid. I know when something hurts and when it doesn't and I know when I do so much that my arm is killing me."

RSI has numerous causes, which is one reason for the confusion about the disorder. Because I have experienced RSI as well as treated it, I know there is hope for you. You are not hysterical, you are not a hypochondriac, and you are not a malingerer. There is effective, conservative treatment that can lead to healing and freedom from pain. This book will help you find the way.

RSI is a general term used to describe a disorder in which people develop symptoms such as pain, numbness, stiffness, and weakness as a result of sustained repetitive work, often done under adverse conditions. These can range from ordinary daily stress to truly bad work setups and work conditions. Usually the pain or other symptoms affect their work and other normal activities. RSI is a widespread illness involving soft tissues of the upper body—nerves, muscles, tendons, ligaments, and blood vessels.

RSI is treatable conservatively for most people using several different approaches, often simultaneously. Posture correction and retraining are often the first steps. Customized physical therapy that includes upper body soft tissue work (we'll get to this procedure of deep massage later in this book) is often required. Strengthening and stretching exercises are also useful, and must be done under supervision. Ergonomic evaluation—the consideration of your work equipment and space—is important, as is training in biomechanics, the proper use of your body to accomplish tasks comfortably and safely. Modifying the way you do things is often necessary, and you can learn to accomplish what you need to do without pain. Finally, both medication and psychological counseling can be useful in controlling pain and healing tissue.

Rarely, surgical intervention is required, but such procedures have their risks as well. In my view, surgery is useful under limited circumstances (e.g., carpal tunnel release surgery). But those patients I have seen after unsuccessful corrective surgeries often become more difficult to treat because of tissue scarring and loss of soft tissue mobility.

RSI by Other Names

Repetitive strain injury is not the only term used to describe this illness. In the scientific community the terms cumulative trauma disorders (CTDs) and repetitive motion disorders are often used. You might be told you have regional arm pain, occupational overuse syndrome (OOS), cervical brachial pain syndrome, work-related musculoskeletal disorder (WRMSD), or upper extremity musculoskeletal disorder (UEMSD). If you are a musician, "overuse syndrome" is often used to describe your problem.

If you are confused, you have a right to be, because the many terms in use reflect the differing and conflicting opinions held by health care professionals.

What Causes RSI?

There are many causes, not all of them obvious. The kind of work you do is perhaps primary, because repetitive keyboard use or repetitive manual activity of any other kind can be a major cause. Long work hours without sufficient breaks and meeting deadlines under stress are also contributors. Poor lighting, poor ventilation, crowding, and other undesirable work environmental issues are additional factors. Even the routine activities of daily life—driving, housekeeping, cooking, gardening, home repairs—can lead to RSI. If you're not sitting or moving correctly, you're damaging yourself repeatedly when you're at work. If your job forces you to work too fast, or to work on irregular schedules, you are at risk. Your physical condition also affects your susceptibility. Poor posture and physical fitness, lack of exercise, deficient diet, and irregular sleep patterns can all be contributory. Stress from family problems, work-related conflicts, or financial affairs can manifest themselves in RSI. Anxiety, depression, fear, and panic also contribute. Sometimes there is a hereditary predisposition to RSI from height, weight, sex, age, or double-jointedness or other anomalies. Medical problems such as diabetes, arthritis, thyroid disease, or hypertension can all make RSI more severe. Finally, smoking, alcohol, and drug use, along with all the other problems such habits bring with them, can also contribute to RSI.

What RSI Isn't

There is at least as much confusion about what RSI isn't as about what it is.

> *It's not carpal tunnel syndrome.* Or at least that's not all it is. Patients often come to me with a self-diagnosis of carpal tunnel syndrome, which most people think is their main problem. Carpal tunnel syndrome (CTS) is one very specific diagnosis, and by no means the major culprit in RSI. In fact, a study of 485 of my most recent patients shows that only 8 percent of them actually had carpal tunnel syndrome. Another study of symptomatic medical secretaries found carpal tunnel syndrome in only 3 percent. Carpal tunnel syndrome is relatively uncommon in keyboard users, and is more often found in workers in heavy industry who do repetitive tasks.

> *It's not regional arm pain.* Another commonly used term for RSI is regional arm pain. Not only does this term imply that the illness is only where the pain is, it also minimizes the seriousness of RSI, putting it into the category of general aches and pains. When a physician tells you that you have regional arm pain, he or she is almost certainly not doing a complete examination. Correct diagnosis depends on a complete upper body physical examination.

> *It's not necessarily a case for the surgeon.* RSI is generally not a condition that requires surgery, although there are advanced conditions that may have progressed beyond conservative treatment. I discuss some of these conditions in chapter 2. It is worth saying here that surgery can often make RSI more difficult to treat conservatively and that you should investigate a conservative therapeutic approach, such as those I outline in this book, before you consider surgery.

RSI is not a mysterious, ill-defined illness. It is not the general aches and pains of growing older. It is not all in the mind.

And it certainly is not a hysterical reaction of bored, lazy, or underperforming workers. In fact, often the hardest-working people are its victims.

In a recent survey of 250,000 businesses employing 101,646,500 people, the U.S. Bureau of Labor Statistics found 276,000 reported RSI cases among office workers, laborers, and fabricators. This number didn't include those working at home, or doing freelance work, or other RSI-affected workers such as dentists, dental hygienists, surgeons, physical and occupational therapists, sign language interpreters, artists, and musicians, to name just a few.

RSI is not the same kind of single-cause occupational illness as asbestosis or black lung disease, but is considered "work-related" because RSI has so many contributing causes.

In my practice, about 60 percent of patients continued their usual work activity even while in pain. Most of them continued to work because they had to keep a steady income or were afraid of losing their jobs. The increasing intensity and chronic nature of their pain are what ultimately brought people to me for evaluation and treatment. Most came in within a year of the onset of their symptoms. Prevention and early intervention are arguably the first lines of defense for all at-risk workers, but because RSI is such a complex illness and is so poorly understood, severe pain and disability precede both the worker's and employer's realization that RSI is the problem. Employers and workers tend to ignore RSI until it hurts both economically and bodily, which means that many people get worse while they work, and continue to work with pain until their problems cause severe injury and can no longer be ignored. These injuries are substantially underreported. And, of course, there are economic consequences as well: money that should be allocated for prevention of injury is lost to higher labor and medical costs after injuries occur.

This book is for the reader who wants to benefit from my clinical experience with RSI and my years of treating people who have it. It was written for people who want to learn how to effectively deal with this illness and are willing to do the work required to get better. You'll learn why RSI is such a complex disorder. You'll learn the causes of RSI and how it affects the body and mind. I'll show you what the latest treatments are, and how to choose the right health professionals to help you carry them out.

I have examined more than four thousand patients with repetitive strain injury. I have learned that RSI is a neuromuscular illness that primarily involves the upper body and that medical specialists often have difficulty diagnosing it. There is no quick fix for RSI—a sad truth that some of you already know. If you want to act, rather than be acted upon, you will have to understand much more about RSI than you now know. There are very few health professionals who have the whole picture on RSI and even fewer who know how to treat it by the latest methods. Remarkably, there is so much misinformation on RSI that you may be learning more about your illness through this book than you have learned from many of your health professionals. Once you take the time to learn some medical facts about the disorder, you can become your own effective advocate in discussing RSI with those who treat you.

1

Understanding RSI

New opinions are always suspected, and usually opposed, without any other reason but because they are not already common.

–John Locke, "An Essay Concerning Human Understanding," 1690

To catch RSI before it becomes a more serious or debilitating illness, it is important to recognize its early signs. There are many risk factors, and every worker should know them. If you understand what happens to the soft tissues as posture deteriorates, you have come a long way toward understanding RSI.

This disorder is insidious–it creeps up on you over a period of weeks, months, or even years. Often patients only recall the day they couldn't take the pain anymore or couldn't continue to work. The process is like a dam that slowly fills with water and then suddenly overflows. In a survey of nearly five hundred of my patients, the most common early signs of RSI were aching or pain in the forearms or hands, numbness and tingling in the hands, weakness in the arms, and spasms or twitching in the forearms. The physician evaluating a person with RSI needs to get a detailed history to assess these symptoms.

Repetitive strain injury is not a diagnosis, but a term used to describe a very complicated, many-faceted soft tissue problem. One reason why RSI is so complicated is that the pain or symptom site is not necessarily where the problem lies. You need a complete physical examination to find out the true cause of the problem.

When you see hundreds of patients, it becomes easier to understand how the many combinations of factors can come together to create RSI. Still, your symptoms may be unique, and unless you get a thorough examination, your physician may not find the cause of your RSI. Without knowing the cause, there can be no effective treatment.

Just as a combination of numbers in the right order is necessary to unlock a safe, so the successful combination in RSI requires the right procedures in the right order. This usually means a complete physical exam, biomechanical and ergonomic intervention, a prescribed treatment program of physical or occupational therapy including a home exercise program, and psychological intervention when needed.

This book devotes a chapter to each of these topics, and our goal is to give you enough information to enable you to get the treatment you need. Essentially, RSI is the result of stress, strain, overuse, and overloading of soft tissues, causing one muscle group to work against another. Sometimes, quirks or anomalies in your anatomy can make you more likely to get injured. How these combine to cause RSI is most easily grasped by beginning with the body's anatomy.

Basic Anatomy

Below are brief descriptions of the most important terms in anatomy that you will come across when you begin seeking help for RSI. Take the time to read this and you will become knowledgeable enough to discuss soft tissue injury with any health professional. Any term not defined here will be found in chapter 2 or the glossary.

The Skeletal System

The skeletal system is the framework that supports the soft tissues. Usually the skeletal system is not directly affected in RSI, with the exception of its most severe complication, late stage reflex sympathetic dystrophy/complex regional pain syndrome

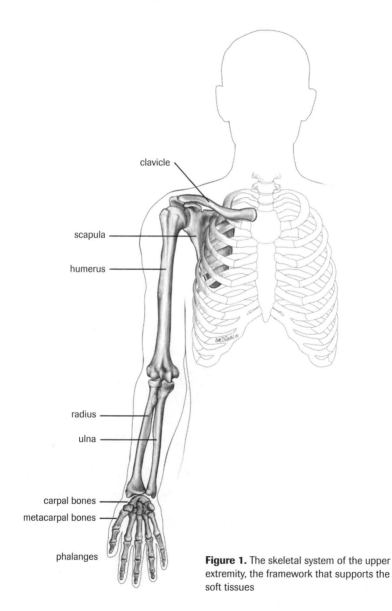

Figure 1. The skeletal system of the upper extremity, the framework that supports the soft tissues

(RSD/CRPS), where bones lose calcium. The ravages of time, arthritis, or injuries to the skeletal system can also make RSI worse.

The Spinal Column

The spinal column has thirty-three individual vertebrae separated by cushioning discs, and it divides into five sections. The upper three sections are movable, while the lower two are fixed. The upper vertebrae connect with one another to form a strong, movable pillar for the support of the head, neck, and trunk. Vertebrae also form a protective ring through which the spinal cord travels to and from the brain. The side arches of two adjacent vertebrae form tunnels (foramina) through which nerves from the spinal cord exit and travel to all parts of the body and return from peripheral sites. If a foramen is partly closed because of injury or arthritic changes, it can squeeze the nerve fiber, causing dysfunction of that nerve. With a slipped disc, the same type of

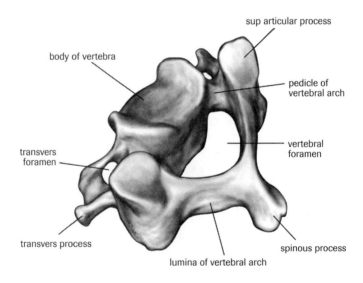

sup articular process

body of vertebra

pedicle of vertebral arch

vertebral foramen

transvers foramen

transvers process

spinous process

lumina of vertebral arch

third cervical vertebra

Figure 2. The spinal column has thirty-three vertebrae separated by cushioning discs. The vertebral foramen is a protective ring through which the spinal cord travels from the brain.

compression occurs where the nerve exits or enters the spinal column. These types of injury are called radiculopathy.

Nerve compression occurs in RSI, usually because of poor posture. After the nerves leave the spinal column they can get caught between tight muscles. This can happen in three areas: in muscles of the neck (scalene muscles), in a space between the collarbone and your first rib, or in a tight space under the smaller pectoral (chest) muscle. When this occurs it is called neurogenic thoracic outlet syndrome (TOS) or brachial plexopathy.

The Shoulder, Back, Neck, and Upper Arm

Your shoulder is the hub around which your arm and hand move. The upper arm bone (humerus), as it rotates in the shoul-

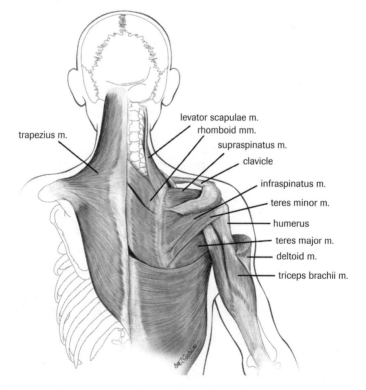

Figure 3. The main musculature of the shoulder and back. The shoulder is the hub around which the arm and hand move.

der socket, forms the most mobile joint in your body. Usually, if posture is poor, the shoulder joint doesn't function properly. When normal shoulder use is lost, the forearm and hand must do more work. Impaired shoulder movement is common in RSI and is a major contributor to symptoms.

The Forearm and the Elbow

As you can see in figure 4, the upper arm and the forearm meet to form the elbow joint. The elbow joint flexes, extends, or rotates the forearm palm up (supination) or palm down (pronation). Repetitive movement can irritate the ulnar nerve at several

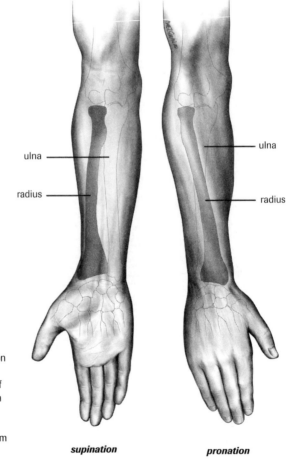

ulna

radius

ulna

radius

Figure 4. Supination and pronation are mainly a function of the elbow, although supination is also controlled by the biceps when the arm is extended.

supination

pronation

points, as it runs from the spinal column through the neck muscles, under the collarbone, then over the first rib and under the small pectoral muscle. The nerve then passes through a bony notch at the elbow joint on its way to the hand. The ulnar nerve normally glides or moves in the neck area. If the nerve is pinched at the neck due to poor posture and tight muscles, then it loses its ability to glide and is pulled tightly through the elbow, causing traction and nerve damage. Think of the ulnar nerve as a long rubber band that is caught and stretched at the neck and that must stretch even tighter as you bend your elbow. This overstretching or traction is called *cubital tunnel syndrome*. The ulnar nerve can also be caught at the wrist, where it is called *ulnar tunnel syndrome*.

A less frequent injury, *radial tunnel syndrome,* happens when another nerve in the arm, the radial nerve, passes by the elbow, then through muscles and ligaments, where it can get compressed. The main difference between these syndromes is that cubital tunnel syndrome happens when the ulnar nerve passes and is stretched around bone, while radial tunnel syndrome happens when the radial nerve passes through tight soft tissue and is squeezed.

The third major nerve in the arm is the median nerve, which can be compressed at the carpal tunnel in the wrist, causing *carpal tunnel syndrome*. This same nerve can also be compressed by muscles below the elbow and is then called *pronator muscle syndrome,* which can be mistaken for carpal tunnel syndrome.

The Wrist

The wrist is a complex structure, and a stable and mobile wrist is important for normal use. Fractures, dislocations, or tears of the ligaments of the wrist bones can lead to instability and pain. So can osteoarthritis of the wrist joints. In patients with RSI, wrist mobility is often impaired because the forearm muscles contract and tighten due to injury.

On the palm side of the wrist, there are nine wrist flexor tendons, which must pass through the same tight carpal tunnel as the

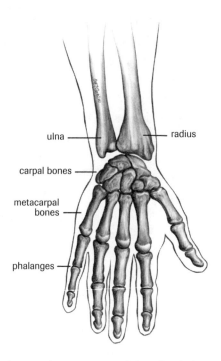

Figure 5. The wrist is a complex structure consisting of an intricate relationship between the forearm and the hand.

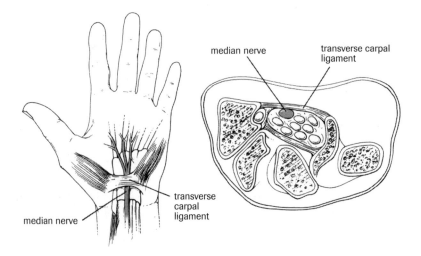

Figure 6. The transverse carpal ligament acts as a pulley guiding the nine flexor tendons of the fingers. The median nerve travels through the same space, making it vulnerable to the injury seen in carpal tunnel syndrome.

median nerve. The combination of shortened muscles in the forearm and tightened tendons at the wrist can cause friction, leading to inflammation, pain and swelling, and carpal tunnel syndrome.

Lying next to the carpal tunnel along the fifth finger side of the wrist is the ulnar tunnel (Guyon's canal). The ulnar nerve can be pinched as it passes by a hooklike bump on the hamate bone of the wrist. This is called *ulnar tunnel syndrome*.

Nerves

Nerves play an important role in RSI because it is the nerves that get trapped or pulled in the injured soft tissues, causing pain, the most common symptom of RSI. Nerves carry pain messages from the site of tissue damage to the brain and have a critical role in muscle regeneration. In the most serious injuries of reflex sympathetic dystrophy/complex regional pain syndrome (RSD/CRPS), the sympathetic branch of the involuntary nervous system, which regulates basic body functions, triggers severe symptoms of pain, temperature and skin color change, swelling, and sweating. And, of course, all this affects motor function.

Muscles

Muscles are the engines that drive all of the movements in the body. For muscles to do their job, they must be well supplied with nutrients and must be connected to functioning nerves. Good performance requires that muscle attachments to tendons, ligaments, and bones are intact and that the joints they move are in good condition. Muscles that are not in balance with other muscles can instigate events that can cause damage to soft tissues. The cascading factors in postural deterioration damage nerves, other soft tissues, and ultimately many other muscles of the body.

Tendons and Ligaments

Tendons are attached between muscle and bone and carry the movement of the muscle to the bone. Tendons are dynamic structures with a rich supply of nerves that permit you to perceive the degree of tension when you move. This perception of tension is called proprioception. Tendons also have specific blood supplies, which can vary in different areas of the tendon. The areas with less blood supply are more likely to be injured when subjected to sustained, repetitive forces.

The term ligament implies that things are tied together, and ligaments do in fact tie muscle to bone, bone to bone, and bone to other soft tissue. But ligaments are also dynamic structures that play an active role in maintaining joint stability and sending signals to the brain regarding their status, another example of proprioception. Ligaments control the limits of joint movements and prohibit exaggerated ones.

Anomalies or Quirks of the Body

Anomalies or quirks are anatomical structures that are not typical in most people. In RSI they cause difficulty by disturbing normal nerve function or making body movement inefficient. The quirk usually known as double-jointedness is one of these. Double-jointedness can be found in the elbow, hands, and fingers, making retraining and therapy more difficult because of the lack of stability in these joints. Double-jointedness is more common in women. People who are double-jointed have to work harder

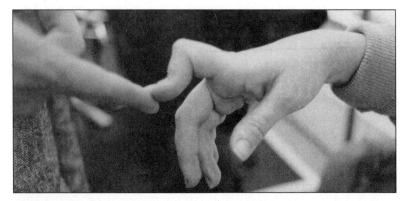

Figure 7. Hyperlaxity, or double-jointedness, in the fingers, makes it more difficult to stabilize the hand while working.

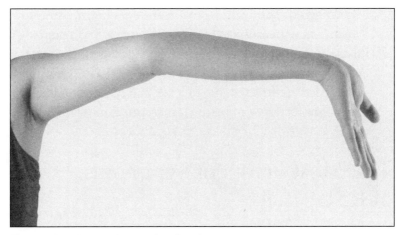

Figure 8. Double-jointedness at the elbow in a young woman

to keep their finger joints stable and curved over their keyboard.

Scalene bands are another anomaly. These are fibrous bands formed between the scalene muscles in the neck. They are only detectable during surgery and are thought to occur in up to 60 percent of the general population. When these bands are present, they create bridges of tissue over which the nerves are stretched and irritated, causing them to stick and not glide as necessary. Thoracic outlet syndrome (TOS), a major problem in RSI, can be caused by these bands.

Anatomy Is Not Always Destiny

There is a saying in medicine that "Anatomy is destiny." In RSI, most anatomical problems can be adequately treated by correcting imbalances in the soft tissues and working around anomalies. With a proper approach to treatment, most of these imbalances are reversible. Steadfast attention to postural retraining, physical and occupational therapy, lifestyle changes, ergonomic and biomechanical modification, and a personal commitment to home exercise programs have proved very effective in my patients.

When the problem is severe and long-term, some soft tissue injuries may be irreversible. When there is severe damage to tissues, healing may never be complete because of scarring, impairment of circulation, or nerve injury. The sooner RSI is diagnosed and treated, the quicker and more complete the comeback. Surgery should be the last resort in most cases.

The Most Frequent Symptoms of RSI

Here are the most common symptoms found in 485 of my patients. Some of the subjects had multiple simultaneous symptoms.

Pain, aching, "spasm" in extremities: 329 (68 percent)

Hand and finger numbness: 55 (11 percent)

Weakness and fatigue: 44 (9 percent)

Tenderness/swelling/inflammation: 43 (9 percent)

Tingling in the fingers: 42 (9 percent)

Tightness/stiffness/rigidity of upper body and neck: 34 (7 percent)

Loss of motor control: 5 (1 percent)

What Your Examination Is Likely to Reveal

Typically, there are several findings for any patient with complaints related to RSI. We'll list the most common here.

Poor Posture

By far the most frequent physical finding in RSI is a characteristic postural misalignment. Typically the head, which weighs about 10 pounds (as much as a bowling ball), is thrust or cantilevered forward and stretches and weakens the upper back and neck muscles, which in turn react by going into a chronic state of contraction. Changes occur in the upper back muscles as they attempt to compensate for this added, constant burden. This cascades into the shoulders, which become hunched and pulled forward. Other muscles in the front of the body such as the scalenes, sternocleidomastoids, and pectoralis minors react by shortening, which sets the stage for nerve damage.

Thoracic Outlet Syndrome

The next most common physical finding is neurogenic thoracic outlet syndrome (TOS). Some people argue that it is more anatomically correct to call it thoracic inlet syndrome (TIS), but we'll stick to the more common term to avoid confusion. As the nerves emerge from the spinal column, they combine into networks. Poor posture causes a soft tissue obstacle as the nerves go through the shortened and tightened scalene muscles. These muscles act like a pair of pincers, squeezing the nerves and causing numbness, tingling, and weakness. This diminishes the ability of the muscles in the extremities to recuperate. In RSI there is a continuing cycle of poor posture leading to nerve damage, which leads to even worse posture and further nerve and muscle compromise. If you understand this process, then you understand how RSI can cascade from minor aches and pains to a totally disabling syndrome. To reverse the process—and it can be reversed for most people—requires your dedication and that of your therapist or therapists.

Reflex Sympathetic Dysfunction

The nerve traction injury of TOS can also involve the sympathetic nerves (involuntary nerves) of the upper body, because the sympathetic nerves become part of this network of nerves in its lower portion near the collarbone. Sympathetic nerve fibers automatically control glands, blood vessels, and smooth muscles. The sympathetic nervous system is part of the autonomic nervous system and therefore is not under our conscious control. Patients' hands are cold and sometimes sweaty, and their perception of pain is usually very high. This condition is called *reflex sympathetic dysfunction*. Rapid intervention is important, because these patients are nearing the more serious complication known as reflex sympathetic dystrophy/complex regional pain syndrome (RSD/CRPS). See chapters 2 and 5 for more on this.

Loss of Shoulder Range of Motion

The shoulder is the most mobile joint in the body. Many of my patients have evidence of shoulder range of motion impairment, which is related to postural misalignment. This restricted shoulder movement becomes painful when extreme movements are attempted. Correcting these conditions is critical because performing activities with limited shoulder movement shifts the workload to the more delicate forearm and hand muscles. Bicipital tendinitis occurs when the tendons of the biceps muscle become irritated in a groove at the shoulder. Postural misalignment is usually associated with this condition.

Cubital Tunnel Syndrome

Cubital tunnel syndrome is far more common than carpal tunnel syndrome. As we follow the ulnar nerve down the arm to the elbow from the neck, we come to an area where the ulnar nerve must pass over a bony cleft or notch at the elbow, which is covered by an arched ligament, creating a tunnel (the cubital tunnel). If the compression at the elbow persists even for just a few months, it can cause a painful condition known as tardy ulnar nerve palsy.

Carpal Tunnel Syndrome

The median nerve runs from the elbow down to the wrist, where it encounters another anatomic tunnel made up of bone and an all-important inelastic roof called the *transverse carpal ligament*. The heavy traffic through this tunnel consists of nine tendons, blood vessels, and the median nerve, which at this point supplies the thumb, index, and middle finger. The transverse carpal ligament (roof) acts like a pulley against which the tendons glide or rub as they move to curl the fingers. The symptoms of carpal tunnel syndrome include sensory complaints such as night pain or numbness and tingling in the first three fingers of the hand. Grasping and pinching are sometimes difficult.

Radial Tunnel Syndrome

Radial tunnel syndrome, also called supinator syndrome, is most likely the result of traction and compression of the radial nerve as it enters a tight canal near the elbow. Basically, the nerve gets caught between two layers of the supinator muscle on its way to the hand. This can result in deep forearm pain followed by gradual fist weakness. This same area is affected in tennis elbow.

Medial Epicondylitis (Golfer's Elbow)

The most common form of tendinitis in persons with RSI is often called golfer's elbow. The *medial epicondyle* is the bony bump at the elbow, where the tendons of the pronator muscles attach. Repetitive pulling on the tendon insertion (where the tendon enters bone) by a damaged or contracted muscle causes inflammation and results in extreme tenderness when pressure is applied.

Lateral Epicondylitis (Tennis Elbow)

Slightly less common than medial epicondylitis in persons with RSI, lateral epicondylitis has similar origins. It occurs in persons who pursue activities with their wrists extended, such as typists, tennis players, and guitarists. Excessive pull at the lateral epicondyle bony bump by tendons can cause inflammation and pain. About 30 percent of the time, tennis elbow and radial tunnel syndrome occur simultaneously, leading some health professionals to call it resistant tennis elbow. When radial tunnel syndrome occurs alone, it can be mistaken for tennis elbow. Only thorough clinical evaluation can clear this up.

DeQuervain's Tenosynovitis

This is a form of tendinitis of the muscles that move the thumb. As the thumb changes direction in use, it can irritate the tendons as they pass through their sheaths, causing inflammation and pain. People who continually lift one thumb to accommodate the

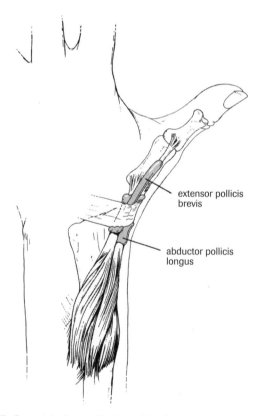

extensor pollicis brevis

abductor pollicis longus

Figure 9. DeQuervain's disease. DeQuervain's disease is a tenosynovitis at the base of the thumb that affects the abductor pollicis longus and the extensor pollicis brevis. It is characterized by the inflammation, thickening, and tenderness of these tendons and their sheaths.

other thumb's use of the space bar, who hit the space bar too forcefully, or who grip their mouse too tightly are at risk for DeQuervain's tenosynovitis.

Myofascial Pain Syndrome

When muscles are injured, they release chemicals that stimulate nerve fibers, causing pain, soreness, and contraction in the hands, forearms, neck, and upper back. With more severe injury, swelling and inflammation occur. Myofascial pain syndrome is a common finding in people with RSI.

Now you have a broad picture of the typical findings in RSI. The next chapter discusses how to help your physician get the diagnosis right.

2

Getting the Diagnosis

Listen to the patient. He's giving you the diagnosis.

−attributed to William Henry Osler (1849–1920)

Over the years, I have become more perplexed about what medical specialty is likely to have physicians trained to evaluate patients with RSI. RSI is a soft-tissue neuromuscular illness, but there is no soft-tissue medical specialty. This illness is difficult and time-consuming to diagnose. I have spent as many as two hours on each first-patient visit to do a full history and complete upper-body examination. Many health care professionals may be less than enthusiastic about doing a complete examination because of time constraints and the complexity of the illness.

Hand surgeons and orthopedists, who often see RSI patients, have been trained to treat illnesses surgically. Generally, RSI is a nonsurgical illness, and though many surgeons recognize this, not all do. Therefore, in choosing a physician, one should look for a specialist who can evaluate an occupational illness with an open mind. After you see your primary care physician, you may be referred to one of the following specialists: an occupational medicine specialist, a hand surgeon, a physiatrist (physical medicine specialist), a neurologist (nerve specialist), a rheumatologist (arthritis specialist), or a pain management specialist. In any case, you want a physician who understands your illness and is able to plan your treatment, refer you to the proper therapists, and follow you through your recovery.

Questions You Need to Get Answered

Does your physician believe RSI exists? This seems rather basic, but there are physicians (and many others) who don't believe this is a disorder at all.

Is your physician listening to you, and is he or she sympathetic? This diagnosis depends heavily on reports from the patient. A health care professional who isn't willing to listen carefully is unlikely to be of much help.

Is your physician willing to spend the time necessary to do a hands-on physical exam? A physical exam is an absolute necessity. If your doctor isn't willing to undertake one, you have to find a doctor who is willing.

Is your physician willing to talk to you about his or her findings, explain them to you, and outline a treatment plan? You have to understand the plan to be able to carry it out. Halfbaked or hasty explanations will not do the trick.

Will your physician advocate for you with your employer and insurance carrier? Not all employers and insurance companies are sympathetic. You need a professional advocate, and your doctor has to be willing to do this for you.

What Your Physician Should Be Looking For

The ultimate goal is to get you adequately examined, diagnosed, and referred for treatment and therapy. This section is not intended for self-diagnosis, but only as a guide to what should be happening when you visit the doctor.

Evaluation begins with a complete medical history. If you can, prior to your first visit write down all you know about how and when your symptoms began; this will be useful to your doctor and will create a common language between the two of you. It is important to include information about your working conditions, type of work, intensity of work, and time spent doing various tasks. Also important is information regarding what kinds of repetitive tasks you engage in at home, at recreation, or at sports.

What you can no longer do as a result of your symptoms is important. Your past medical history, any illness or accidents you have had including car accidents, medications you are taking, your sleeping, eating, and exercise habits, and any eyesight problems should also be included. Don't forget to mention any stress you are under, from any source, and how it may be affecting your emotions.

Specific work information will be needed about keyboard use, input devices, seating, and monitor placement, plus environmental factors such as lighting, glare, ventilation, and crowding. How and when you use your laptop computer and input devices, as well as phone use and any difficulty you have with handwriting, are also important. Photographs or videotapes of you at your workstation are helpful.

This is the kind of information you must provide so the physician can complete his or her history. Certain basic diagnostic and lab tests that are typically done by your primary care physician should be part of your history package.

To guide you, on the next few pages is a questionnaire I ask my patients to complete before they come to our facility.

Patient Questionnaire

Patient name _____

Age _____   Sex M _____   F _____

Occupation _____   Height _____   Weight _____

Hand dominance R ____ L ____ Eye dominance R ____ L ____

General health history: Please list any past or current health problems, surgeries, or upper-body injuries with dates.

_____

_____

Current medications _____

_____

Sleep well? ____ Yes ____ No

Appetite good? ____ Yes ____ No

Do you smoke? ____ Yes ____ No ____#/day

Do you exercise? ____ Never ____ Occasionally ____ Regularly

(describe) _____

Current problem:

Chief complaint (current symptoms) _____

_____

Date of onset _____   Initial symptoms _____
Description of circumstances

When are symptoms most prevalent ____ A.M. ____ P.M.
  ____ During work ____ After work ____ Constant

What doctors have you seen for this problem? (If more than two, please list on the back)

Date _____   M.D. name _____   Specialty _____

Diagnosis _____   Treatment _____

(continued)

Date _____ M.D. name _____ Specialty _____

Diagnosis _____ Treatment _____

Please list any tests performed, and provide copies of results (e.g., EMG, MRI, blood work, X-rays) _____

_____

_____

Did you ever wear splints? ___ No ___ Yes _____ At work
___ To sleep   Duration? _____

Do you drop things frequently?   ___ No ___ Yes

Had physical or occupational therapy for this problem?
___ No ___ Yes Duration? _____

Have activities of daily living been affected? ___ No ___ Yes

___ Driving   ___ Doing dishes   ___ Opening doors
___ Opening jars   ___ Carrying bags   ___ Writing
___ Dressing   ___ Holding books/turning pages
___ Vacuuming   ___ Using scissors

Other _____

Computer workload: Average hours at keyboard per day _____

___ Straight input   ___ Editing   ___ Intellectual use
___ Bingework   ___ Mixed use   ___ Writing
___ Phone   ___ Filing   ___ Mouse
___ Voice-activated   ___ V.A. type

How often do you take breaks? _____

  Duration? _____

What do you do on a break? _____

Workstation Setup:

Type of keyboard _____

Type of mouse _____
  Is it at keyboard height? ___ Yes ___ No

(continued)

31

Patient Questionaire (continued)

Adjustable chair ___ Yes ___ No
  ___ Seat pan tilt ___ Lumbar support

Adjustable desk ___ Yes ___ No ___ Keyboard tray

Adjustable monitor ____ In front of keyboard ____ To left
  ____ To right

Copyholder ____ None ____ Left ____ Right

Frequently on the phone while typing or writing? ___ Yes
  ___ No

Do you use a headset? ___ Yes ___ No

More than one workstation? ___ Yes ___ No
  Describe _____

General work conditions (lighting, ventilation, stress factor,
  etc.) ___ Good ___ Fair ___ Poor

Have you reported your symptoms to your employer? ___ Yes
  ___ No

What was the response? ___ Good (open to changes)
  ___ Noncommittal ___ Hostile

Other intensive use of hand ___ Gardening
  ___ Musical instrument: _____
  ___ Handcrafts ___ Other _____
  Hrs. per week _____

Injury: On the job ___ Date _____ Auto accident ___
Date _____

  Sports ___ Date _____ Other ___ Date _____

Additional comments _____

_____

The Pain Pictogram

Since pain is the main reason why people seek help, a pain pictogram like the one below is very useful to graphically show your pain pattern to your physician and therapists. Many patients have told me that filling out the pictogram is the first visualization they have of their pain sites. By grading your pain level on a scale from 1 to 10 in each area on the pictogram you will give perspective to the examining physician about your condition.

The Physical Examination

Most of the findings in RSI are revealed via a comprehensive physical examination. Because medicine has become highly specialized, physicians are losing their hands-on clinical skills,

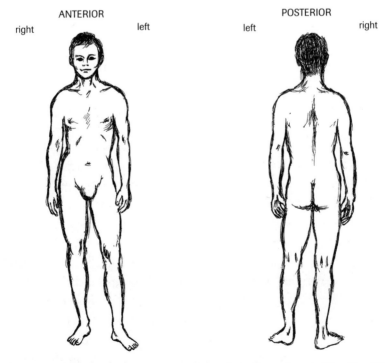

Figure 10a and Figure 10b. Patients are asked to mark the figures for pain (*), aching (**), burning (•), stiffness (+), and numbness (++).

and a general physical examination is less frequently performed than in the past. Modern-day medicine encourages reliance on laboratory studies and tests to make diagnostic decisions. In RSI, however, a negative EMG or MRI may not reflect the positive findings seen in the clinical part of the examination. Some testing is necessary in certain circumstances, but no test can substitute for a complete upper-body physical exam. The useful tests are outlined later in this section.

Physicians are beginning to recognize the importance of the hands-on physical exam. The National Board of Medical Examiners (NBME) and the Federation of State Medical Boards (FSMB) are pushing for a Clinical Skills Assessment Examination (CSAE) as part of the U.S. Medical Licensing Examination. While groups representing medical students are theoretically in support of the need for enhanced clinical skills, they have objected to the cost and inconvenience of taking such a test. Ironically, it is the high cost of medical education that has pushed many students into specialty medicine, where the financial rewards are usually greater. This has resulted in fewer students moving into primary care, where a clinically skilled physician could actually help avoid incurring many of the high costs associated with specialty care. This is especially true in RSI. In my view, the single factor having the most impact on the cost and quality of care in the diagnosis and treatment of RSI is the lack of clinical skills of the physician. Even if the clinician had these skills, he would be thwarted by the lack of financial incentive to perform the kind of examination required to carry out focused treatment. This has also resulted in patients, in order to seek a cure, visiting many physicians in a variety of specialties, leading to mounting costs and a large number of unnecessary surgeries and other treatments. It is encouraging that some attention is being focused on improving the clinical skills of students and practitioners.

The objective of the physical examination is to provide as accurate a set of clinical diagnoses as possible. The following section identifies areas of your upper body that need to be examined. We will get to more specific findings later in this chapter. The progression in an upper-body exam usually begins with the hands and progresses up to the shoulders, upper back, neck, and head. There are so many items in a clinical RSI examination that I always use a printed protocol to guide me through the examination.

Hands

The hands are examined for finger length, double-jointedness, swelling, tenderness, tremor, skin color, and condition. Temperature changes, especially cold hands and sweaty palms, are often overlooked and are important, as they indicate abnormality of the involuntary nervous system. Contraction of the muscles of the hand, causing cupping of the palm when the hand is at rest, confirms that there are nerve and muscle fiber changes. DeQuervain's disease is verified by Finkelstein's test. This test is performed by having the patient make a fist with the thumb placed inside the palm. The wrist is then laterally flexed toward the fifth finger (ulnar deviation), thus stretching the thumb tendons, which, if inflamed, will elicit pain at the base of the thumb. This pain indicates a positive diagnosis. The hands are also checked for the presence of ganglion cysts, trigger fingers, and functional anomalies such as Linburg's tendon, where tendons of the thumb and index finger are abnormally attached. Finally, the finger strength (pinch test) is performed. This is done with an instrument called a dynamometer, which measures the strength of the fingers in various positions.

Wrists

Wrist evaluation should focus on range-of-motion testing in flexion (wrist bent downward) and extension (wrist bent upward). If loss of range of wrist motion is found, it usually suggests that you have shortened forearm muscles. Neurologic testing for carpal tunnel syndrome and ulnar tunnel syndrome is performed. Tapping over the nerve to elicit tingling (Tinel's test) is helpful for detecting nerve irritability. In carpal tunnel syndrome we look for muscle wasting. Phelan's test is recommended—this increases pressure on the median nerve by bending the wrist in flexion for a minute, and producing numbness. If there is any doubt, electromyography should be performed to document median nerve compression. If the muscle reaction is delayed by more than four milliseconds, the test is positive. Yet negative results do not rule out carpal tunnel syndrome. Muscle testing is useful especially for ruling out median nerve compression farther up the arm (pronator syndrome) or anterior interosseous syndrome.

Ulnar tunnel syndrome is diagnosed in a similar fashion, checking for swelling, particularly that caused by a ganglion. Loss of motor function is more common in ulnar tunnel syndrome than in carpal tunnel syndrome. Nerve conduction velocity studies can be helpful in detecting compression between the wrist and the hand muscles.

Forearms

Forearms are examined for muscle soreness, tenderness, and evidence of muscle tightness. If these muscles are tight, they "jump" like plucked violin strings as the examiner runs a thumb across them. Grip strength is tested by using an instrument called the Jamar dynamometer, which records grip power in pounds per square inch. The instrument can be adjusted for smaller or larger hands.

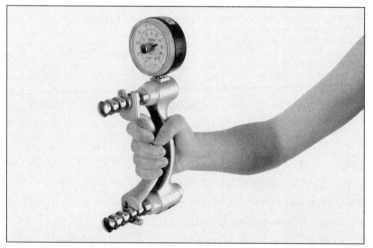

Figure 11. The Jamar Dynamometer for testing grip strength

Elbows

Elbows are tested for range of motion, which should be measured in extension (straight out), flexion (bent at elbow), supination (palms up), and pronation (palms down). Elbows are also tested for tendinitis and nerve impingement by palpation, tapping (Tinel's test), or electromyography.

The "carrying angle," which is the angle between the humerus and ulna bones, is examined (see chapter 9). This is impor-

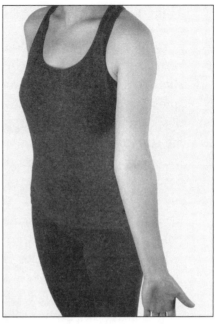

Figure 12. This woman's carrying angle at the elbow is increased.

tant because your carrying angle determines how your arms are positioned at the keyboard. People with a carrying angle greater than ten degrees probably need an angled or split keyboard.

Shoulders

Shoulder examination is extremely important but often neglected. Shoulder examination should include testing for range of motion, which is measured for internal rotation, external rotation, abduction, adduction, forward flexion, forward extension, and horizontal flexion and extension. The shoulder is also examined for evidence of bursitis, bicipital tendinitis, instability, impingement, and rotator cuff strain or tear.

Rounded shoulders, often combined with a protruding neck or head, can lead to muscle imbalance that will compress and stretch nerves. This is the first step in a cascade that leads to the problems encountered in the forearms and hands of people with RSI.

Posture

Postural misalignment is one of the pivotal findings in persons with RSI. It is essential to check for shoulder protraction (round shoulders). Stiffness or immobility of the cervical or thoracic spine can frequently be found—they become immobile because of spasm of the muscles supporting the spinal column. Protruding scapulas (winging) may be observed because of weakness of the muscles that stabilize the shoulder blades. This usually occurs if the patient is deconditioned, or the nerves supplying the scapular stabilizers are compromised. Finally, upper trapezius muscles adjacent to the neck tighten as a compensating reaction, since these muscles are recruited to do the work of the failing upper back muscles. The road back will mean that posture should be corrected and poorly functioning muscles strengthened and brought back to full activity.

Scoliosis, or a crooked spine, is often hereditary, but should be looked for since it can contribute to muscle imbalance.

Neck

The neck is checked for range of motion for flexion, extension, rotation and lateral flexion, and a forward head position. You are checked for pain, which occurs when thumb pressure is exerted at the base of the neck above and below the collarbone (mechanical allodynia). Neurologic tests such as the Roos (Elevated Arm Stress Test) test, Wright's test, and mechanical allodynia for thoracic outlet syndrome are performed.

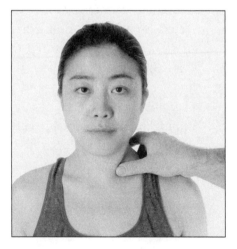

Figure 13. Thumb pressure testing for mechanical allodynia

Tests

Often insurance companies and lawyers may demand what they consider "objective" tests such as EMGs or MRIs, even though many of the physical exam tests are also objective. Patients may urge that tests be done to reassure themselves that a catastrophic illness is not lurking in their bodies. It is up to the examining physician to determine if and when they should be done. Speaking to patients about these findings is important.

Here are some of the tests that might be ordered. Many do not have a direct relationship to RSI, and this list is by no means comprehensive.

Roos Test

Also known as the EAST test, elevated arm stress test, this involves placing the patient's arms in the "hold-up position" for three minutes. It is a reliable test for bringing out symptoms such as weakness, numbness, and tingling in people who have neurogenic thoracic outlet syndrome.

Wright's Test

This has a similar rationale. It involves extending both arms straight up, which produces symptoms by stretching or pulling on the nerves in the neck, or possibly a loss or a diminution of the wrist pulse.

Mechanical Allodynia

Allodynia means that pain occurs from a stimulus that ordinarily would not produce pain. Mechanical allodynia involves the therapist pressing on a muscle and its nerves with the pad of the thumb. The impaired tissue releases pain-producing substances helpful in diagnosis.

Other Tests

Cervical radiculopathy (see pages 55–56) is suspected when pain is elicited by applying downward pressure on the flexed neck. If pain is elicited, further tests such as cervical spine X-rays, CT scans, and/or MRI would be indicated. Cervical radiculopathy as a cause of neck pain is far less common than brachial plexopathy. In other words, in people with RSI, the soft tissues of the neck are more likely to cause nerve trouble than the bony or cartilaginous structures. With increasing age, radiculopathy becomes more common.

Muscle Testing

It is also useful to test muscle strength to find the areas where weakness occurs because of nerve and/or muscle damage. In TOS this muscle damage and weakness will usually be found in the hands and forearms.

Clinical Nerve Testing

Look for Tinel's sign, where the physician taps on the nerves with his fingers—at the elbow or the wrist, for example—to see if you feel tingling or pain. Test for deep tendon reflexes with a reflex hammer. Perform the Semmes-Weinstein monofilament test for sensory loss. Test for two-point discrimination for nerve progressive status.

Diagnostic and Lab Tests

I stress the importance of a complete physical examination for people suspected of having RSI. Certain basic diagnostic and lab tests that are typically done by your primary care physician should be part of an RSI examination. For a number of reasons, the examining physician may feel compelled to perform additional tests. If an accompanying or contributing illness is suspected, such tests can aid in the diagnosis.

Biofeedback

Biofeedback furnishes the examiner and the patient with information on the state of bodily processes such as skin temperature and heart rate through the use of a machine with electrodes attached to the body. The test usually involves an auditory or visual response through which the patient can gain some voluntary control over the bodily process. Biofeedback is also useful in the treatment of reflex sympathetic dysfunction as well as RSI and low back syndrome, and can provide feedback during biomechanical retraining sessions.

Bone Densitometry

This test is used to determine loss of bone mass in conditions such as osteoporosis or osteopenia.

Bone Scan

Scan is a short term for scintiscan. It maps the bones by illustrating the concentration of gamma rays emitted by an injected isotope that seeks out bone. Osteoporosis and bone tumors can be detected by this technique. Scintiscans can be obtained for other body organs when organ-specific isotopes are used.

Computerized Tomography (CT Scan)

Computerized tomography has replaced plain X-rays in a number of different areas. It has revolutionized diagnostic radiology. CT scans utilize low doses of X-rays and then computerize the absorption of X-rays by tissues such as the brain skull and spinal fluid to create images of these tissues that resemble actual slices through the body. Contrast medium is sometimes injected to enhance the quality of the image.

Electrocardiography (ECG)

ECG is a test that measures the electrical activity of the heart muscle. It is useful in distinguishing the chest pain of heart disease from that of TOS, and detecting irregularities of heart rhythm.

Electromyography (EMG)

Like an electrocardiogram, EMG measures the electrical activity of muscle. Normal muscle is electrically silent at rest. By inserting a needle into muscle and observing the quality and quantity of action potentials that occur when muscle is contracted, deviations from the norm can be detected. A refinement of this technique is used for demonstrating focal dystonia (writer's cramp), which is sometimes seen in musicians and typists. Here a thin wire is inserted into individual muscle bundles to demonstrate an abnormal muscle contraction pattern. The latter technique is used primarily as a research tool.

Electroneurography (Nerve Conduction Velocity or NCV)

This test is used in RSI patients to demonstrate compression of a nerve such as the median nerve in carpal tunnel syndrome or ulnar nerve traction at the elbow in cubital tunnel syndrome. In these syndromes, slowing of the electrical impulse along the motor nerve fiber is seen. It is less useful in demonstrating the soft tissue nerve compression in the neck caused by thoracic outlet syndrome, because of the number and density of the nerve roots. Since TOS is clinically so common in RSI, a negative result in NCV testing can divert the physician from this important diagnosis. Because of variability in standards, this test is only as good as the person performing and interpreting it.

Infrared Camera Analysis

The infrared camera allows the examiner to detect real-time changes in skin temperature during movement. Presently very few facilities have this equipment. In the future, it may prove extremely useful to confirm the diagnosis of reflex sympathetic dysfunction (RSD) or complex regional pain syndrome (CRPS).

Magnetic Resonance Imaging (MRI)

This truly revolutionary technique does not require X-ray exposure. MRI uses a magnetic field to obtain a detailed picture of the body's soft tissues. It is useful for investigating the soft tissue injury that characterizes RSI. If the patient has a cardiac monitor, pacemaker, or surgical clips in the brain, a CT scan must be done instead.

Plethysmography

This test measures the intensity of pulse waves in various parts of the body. It is useful in detecting arterial compression when the patient changes position, as might occur in thoracic outlet syndrome, when blood vessels are compressed.

Positive Emission Tomography (PET Scan)

This technique is performed in nuclear medicine facilities and is not available in all hospitals. Like CTs and MRIs it involves "slicing" or cross-sectional data-gathering. At present it is specifically used to investigate the brain, heart, and lungs. It is not a frequently used test in RSI patients except where there is suspicion of a coexisting illness.

Surface Electromyography (Surface EMG)

This technique uses a number of electrodes placed over muscle groups to analyze muscle contraction. It is also a useful biofeedback tool.

Thermography

Thermography uses infrared imaging to locate skin temperature differences in various parts of the body. It is considered important in the management of chronic pain and in the diagnosis of reflex sympathetic dysfunction and complex regional pain syndrome. It is available in only a few facilities. Some centers have an improved version capable of computer-assisted thermography.

X-rays (Radiographs)

X-rays are electromagnetic vibrations of short wavelengths. They penetrate some substances more readily than others and act on photographic film. They are useful in RSI to detect bone problems such as osteoporosis, fractures, and anomalies. X-ray analysis is less useful for evaluating soft-tissue problems.

Vibrometry

This test is used to test the sensitivity of peripheral nerves that might have been damaged by a vibration injury. Generally, computer users don't get vibration syndrome, although recent studies have shown evidence that this does occur in some. If you have been engaged in other activities involving vibration, this test can also be helpful.

Blood Tests

The following are blood tests that are done to rule out various illnesses, also listed here, that might be contributing to RSI symptoms:

Chemical profile: cholesterol, triglycerides, and liver and kidney functions, among others

Complete blood count (CBC): anemia, infection, and disorders such as leukemia, lymphoma, Hodgkin's disease, and lupus

Erythrocyte sedimentation rate (ESR): infection, arthritis, arteritis, and anemia

Blood sugar: diabetes mellitus

Cholesterol and triglycerides: coronary artery disease

Serum iron and iron binding capacity: anemia and iron transport diseases

Rheumatoid factor: arthritis

Antinuclear antibodies (ANA): lupus, connective tissue disorders, scleroderma, rheumatoid arthritis

Thyroid hormone levels and thyroid stimulating hormone (TSH): thyroid disease, hyperthyroidism, hypothyroidism

Electrolytes (potassium, sodium, calcium chloride, phosphorus): various metabolic deficiencies

Profiles of Injury: The Significant Findings in RSI

To get a broader picture of RSI it is helpful to look at a large group of RSI patients. This section profiles the findings found in RSI patients that I have seen in the past few years of my practice and covers the most significant diagnoses I found in these patients.

In my group of RSI patients, 70 percent used the computer for most of their workday. About 25 percent were musicians who were injured primarily from playing their instruments. The remainder were in professions where repetitive tasks were common. When first seen, almost 60 percent were working full-time despite symptoms. Sixteen percent had lost their jobs due to RSI, and 1 percent were receiving disability payments. That so many people in pain were still at work suggests that the stereotype of the malingering employee should be rethought and that many workers' injuries are not reported to the workers' compensation system.

How RSI Begins

In RSI, early recognition and early treatment mean quicker recovery. In 56 percent of my injured patients, aching, pain, and "spasms" in the extremities were the first signs of RSI. Patients generally used the term "spasms" to describe twitches, while a few used this term to describe muscle tightness. Ten percent also noted hand and finger numbness, while weakness, fatigue tingling, and stiffness occurred in about 6 to 7 percent. Less frequently, tenderness of the muscles and vague discomfort were reported. About 18 percent did not recall details of their first symptoms. RSI usually develops slowly, so it is understandable that some people will not recall the early signs of their illness. However, most of my patients came to our facility within a year of the onset of their first symptoms. Increase in pain is the principal reason why people with RSI finally seek care. In some cases, a marked increase in numbness and tingling, weakness, and muscle tenderness and swelling is the trigger for seeking help.

Postural Misalignment

The most frequent physical finding in patients seeking care for RSI is postural misalignment. I found this in almost 80 percent of my patients. Generally, as we age, our posture deteriorates, an outcome even more likely if we've spent years hunched over a keyboard or performing a variety of other repetitive tasks without preventive upper-body conditioning. In postural misalignment, the head, thrust forward, stretches and weakens the upper back and neck muscles. The shoulders are hunched and pulled forward, and muscles in the front of the body react by shortening, setting the stage for nerve damage. As nerves emerge from the spinal column (where they might be compressed by a disc or a bone spur, causing radiculopathy), they combine into networks called the cervical plexus and brachial plexus.

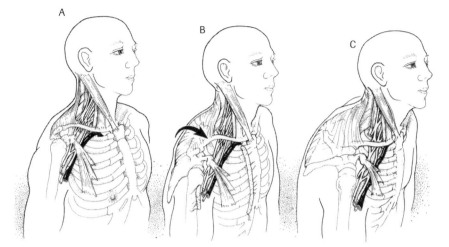

Figure 14. Progressive postural distortion/decompensation with neurovascular compression. A: Normal resting posture. B: Shoulder protraction beginning; sternomastoid muscles are shortening, drawing head anteriorly and inferiorly. C: Advanced deformity with adaptive shortening of scalene and smaller pectoral muscles. Note narrowed costoclavicular space as well (ribs 1 through 5 have been relatively elevated). Neurovascular compression is evident at all three sites.

Neurogenic Thoracic Outlet Syndrome (TOS)

In this syndrome, nerves encounter a series of tight spots as they travel from the neck to the arms and hands. The brachial plexus nerves encounter what is their first soft-tissue obstacle in the scalene muscles. Two of the three scalenes act like a pair of pincers when they are shortened and tightened and can squeeze the brachial plexus nerves. Since the scalene muscles are also attached to the upper ribs, they can affect breathing if they are tight. Stretching these tightened muscles to relieve pressure on nerves is a basic component of treatment and should be accompanied by breathing exercises. About 70 percent of RSI patients will have this diagnosis.

Once the nerves emerge from between the scalene muscles, the next tight spot they encounter is between the collarbone (clavicle) and the first rib. With the tightened scalene muscles pulling the first rib up, the space between the collarbone and the first rib narrows, to become another area of potential pressure on the nerve bundle as it descends to the arm. At this point, the nerve bundle is joined by vascular structures and encounters another tight spot as it goes under the pectoralis minor muscle along the upper chest. With postural misalignment, these muscles will be shortened, tightened, and painful to pressure (see figure 14). Occasionally the tightened pectoralis minor muscles can compress the large arm artery (subclavian artery) so that when an arm is raised above the heart, a loss of pulse occurs. This can usually be remedied by a course of stretching and postural retraining. If nerves are compressed in any of the above-mentioned areas, the nerve bundle will lose its capacity to slide, undergoing pulling or traction as you move your arms. This is a very common injury, which I have found in 70 percent of my patients.

A number of anatomic quirks, which we may be born with, can predispose us to developing TOS. The most common are scalene muscles that are enlarged or attached too far forward on the first rib. Sometimes fibrous bands of tissue can bridge the scalene muscles, resulting in a tethering of these nerves, which then cannot glide as they should. Between 30 and 60 percent of the general population have these bands. Bony abnormalities such as an extra rib are less common anatomic quirks. People with a long neck and drooping shoulders can also be at risk for TOS. Whiplash injuries appear to cause TOS in certain cases, and migraine headaches can accompany TOS. In my experience this is a neglected cause of migraines.

Because the brachial and cervical nervous networks involve so many different nerve branches, and encounter so many soft-tissue obstacles related to poor posture, injury to various areas of these nerves can present different symptoms. Knowledge of these symptoms can help the examining physician locate the site of nerve compression or traction.

Superior trunk injury causes pain radiating into the shoulder down the arm and along the central portion of the shoulder blade (see figure 15). This can cause swelling in the face and neck as well as atypical severe migraine headaches not responsive to the usual migraine medications. This is an easily missed diagnosis, as it is often confused with ordinary migraine headaches.

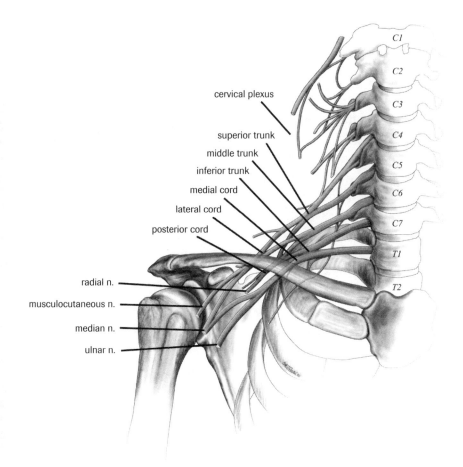

Figure 15. The cervical plexus and brachial plexus are the keys to understanding RSI and its pain patterns.

Medial cord injury causes pain in the front portion of the neck, which radiates down the forearm to the fourth and fifth fingers.

Inferior trunk injury causes dull aching pain in the forearm, with tingling or burning of the fourth and fifth fingers, as well as weakness of the thumb muscles and intrinsic hand muscles. This lesion is the most common form of neurogenic thoracic outlet syndrome.

Lateral cord injury causes severe pain in the area below the collarbone and tingling of the thumb, index, middle finger, and occasionally the palm. In this case, chest wall pain can be misdiagnosed as a cardiac event such as a heart attack.

Posterior cord injury causes tingling or burning over the triceps muscle of the arms as well as the tennis elbow area (lateral epicondyle). Sometimes tingling and burning are felt in the forearm, thumb, index, and middle fingers.

TOS traction injuries can also cause reflex sympathetic dysfunction. This involves the sympathetic nerves of the upper body because they become part of the nerve network near the collarbone. The sympathetic nervous system is part of the autonomic or involuntary nervous system and is not under our conscious control. Sympathetic nerve fibers control glands, blood vessels, and smooth muscle. About 20 percent of the patients I examined with TOS had manifestations of "sympathetic overdrive." Their hands were cold and sometimes sweaty, and their pain level was increased. This condition is usually called reflex sympathetic dysfunction. Here, rapid intervention is important. Muscles and joints should not be immobilized with splints, and an aggressive physical therapy program should be undertaken along with an appropriate medication. This condition may lead to the more severe complication known as reflex sympathetic dystrophy (RSD), which is now called complex regional pain syndrome (CRPS).

Failure to recognize or improper treatment of reflex sympathetic dysfunction can develop into reflex sympathetic dystrophy/complex regional pain syndrome (RSD/CRPS). It is critical to realize that any soft-tissue injury can result in RSD/CRPS, a severe evolutionary phase of sympathetic overdrive. The injury can be caused by excessive typing or other repetitive movements; trauma, such as getting your hand or arm caught in a door; or occasionally from operations, such as a carpal tunnel release or other surgery. Early and aggressive treatment is essential.

RSD/CRPS is usually divided into three stages, as suggested by neurologist Robert J. Schwartzman, M.D.: stage I, in which there is increased sensitivity to touch and heat stimuli; stage II, in which symptoms increase in intensity and pain spreads; and stage III, in which pain can spread to lower extremities or the other side of the upper body.

Two patients I recently saw illustrate the need for the examining physician to be alert. Unfortunately, in both cases they came in six months after their precipitating episode, and both were in stage II, when treatment measures are far less successful.

A. B. was a fifty-year-old woman, a hardworking office supervisor who performed her tasks with no obvious difficulty. She did have a history of Lyme disease, for which she received antibiotics over a six-year period. One day, as she was going through a doorway, her hand got caught in the push bar of the door. She pulled away abruptly. She sustained both a crush injury to the hand and a pulling or traction injury to the brachial plexus. Both of these injuries were potentially precipitating events for RSD/CRPS. She was disabled because of the delay in her treatment caused by the late diagnosis.

The same was true for C. F., a sanitation worker whose hand was injured while he was at work. He, too, sustained a crush injury to his hand and a traction injury to the brachial plexus. His pain was so severe that a light touch to his skin produced paroxysms of pain. The lesson here is that the diagnosis of this disorder needs to be made early. This requires a high degree of suspicion by the examining physician, who should obtain the necessary information from a thorough history and physical exam.

As to the illness progress, visible tissue changes occur in the upper extremities and include thickened and shiny skin, brittle and cracked nails, contracted joints, and calcium loss in the bones. In the later stages of evolution, patients with RSD/CRPS become weak in the affected muscles, which develop spasm, increased irritability, and exaggerated tremor. At this stage it also is difficult for RSD/CRPS patients to initiate movement.

Therapeutic intervention with physical therapy and certain medications should be started immediately with the assistance of a pain management specialist, who might enlist a more aggressive approach to treatment, such as nerve blocks, which are most effective in the first six months. See chapter 5 for more details.

Cubital tunnel syndrome occurs in more than 60 percent of the people I examined. The ulnar nerve runs from the neck to the elbow, where it must pass under a bony cleft or notch through a tunnel roofed over by an arched ligament at the elbow. As the elbow is bent, greater pull or traction is exerted on the nerve. If the ulnar nerve is locked in place at the neck, as occurs in TOS, then bending the elbow will distress the nerve at this second point; some call this a double crush. This is why I recommend use of the hands and forearms with the elbow open instead of at a right angle when using the keyboard. Tardy ulnar nerve palsy occurs when the ulnar nerve remains injured for a long time, causing muscle weakness. A ganglion cyst in the cubital tunnel is another possible reason for ulnar nerve compression.

Ulnar tunnel syndrome (Guyon's canal syndrome) describes yet another potential area of compression of the ulnar nerve; this occurs at the wrist in a tunnel adjacent to the carpal tunnel. We found this syndrome in about 10 percent of our patients. Symptoms include pain, numbness, and tingling in the third, fourth, and fifth fingers; these symptoms are aggravated by bending the hand upward at the wrist (wrist extension).

There are many potential causes of ulnar tunnel syndrome, ranging from anatomic abnormalities to fracture of the hamate bone (a wrist bone), to riding bicycles with awkward handlebars, to arthritis. In typists and musicians, this may be due to repetitive wrist extension coupled with windshield-wiperlike bending of the hands at the wrist.

Median Nerve Injury

Pronator Teres Muscle Syndrome

Here the median nerve, which also derives from the brachial plexus, is squeezed between the two heads of the pronator teres muscle below the elbow. This is the muscle that moves the forearm and hand into the palms-down position used in typing and piano playing. The median nerve winds its way through several forearm muscles before entering the carpal tunnel. Since the median nerve has a branch that goes over the wrist before entering the carpal tunnel, injury to that nerve segment can cause sensory disturbances over both surfaces of the hand. In pronator syndrome, numbness of the whole palm is the important distinguishing feature; in carpal tunnel syndrome, usually just the thumb, forefinger, and middle finger are involved.

There are many possible causes of pronator syndrome. Trauma and muscle inflammation of repetitive movement probably play a major role in what we see in computer users. We have found this syndrome in 6 percent of our patients.

Carpal Tunnel Syndrome

It is very important to distinguish the symptoms of carpal tunnel syndrome from those of pronator syndrome to avoid inappropriate surgery. We hear a lot about carpal tunnel syndrome, which is often misused as a synonym for RSI. Although EMGs and NCVs are considered to be the diagnostic "gold standard," research has shown that the most reliable way to diagnose carpal tunnel syndromes (CTS) is a pictogram of the hand filled out by the patient. Actually, I have found this syndrome in about 8 percent of my patients, and have rarely sent anyone with CTS for a surgical release unless there was atrophy of the muscles at the base of the thumb and the palm (the thenar eminence), which indicates more advanced damage involving the motor branch of the nerve.

The symptoms of carpal tunnel syndrome include sensory complaints in the hands and fingers such as night pain, numbness, and tingling. Grasping and pinching are sometimes difficult. The traffic through the carpal tunnel consists of nine finger flexor tendons, blood vessels, and the median nerve, which supplies the thumb, index, and middle finger (see figure 6). The transverse carpal ligament, or roof of the carpal tunnel, acts like a pulley against which the tendons glide or rub as they move to curl the fingers. Picture a fishing rod with rings through which the fishing line runs; remove a ring and the line "bowstrings" to the next ring. This is what happens if the transverse carpal ligament is cut in the carpal tunnel release operation. This places tension on the next set of pulleys, which are located in the fingers. Trigger finger results from the increased friction and inflammation in these tendons, which can develop nodules or become inflamed and swollen, causing the tendons to get caught in the finger pulleys when the fingers are flexed. Surgery may be necessary to correct trigger finger.

In my experience, patients with carpal tunnel syndrome almost always sustain a loss of normal wrist range of motion. This is probably the result of the forearm muscles shortening due to overuse, combined with a loss of the capacity to regenerate muscle. Repetitive wrist motion results in a rise in pressure in the tunnel. Gentle, gradual range-of-motion exercises of the wrist, coupled with forearm massage and correction of ergonomic problems, can in most cases obviate the need for surgery.

While carpal tunnel syndrome is regarded as a median nerve compression problem, in addition to the median nerve, nine flexor tendons of the fingers run through the carpal tunnel. Since virtually all those with carpal tunnel syndrome lose range of motion in their wrists because of shortened forearm muscles, these shortened muscles can be the cause of the greater friction in the carpal tunnel. The increase in carpal tunnel pressure also diminishes blood supply to the tendons and the median nerve. Stretching and forearm muscle massage and strengthening are important to correct this condition. The question of splints— when and if to use them—is discussed in chapter 5.

Radial Nerve Injury

Radial Tunnel Syndrome

Also called supinator syndrome, this is most likely the result of both traction and compression of the radial nerve as it enters a tight canal at the elbow, which is sometimes roofed over by a tendinous arch called the arcade of Fröhse. The nerve gets caught between two layers of the supinator muscle on its way to the hand. This can result in deep forearm pain, followed by gradual fist weakness and local pain on pressing of the lateral epicondyle (bony prominence in the elbow).

Radial tunnel syndrome occurs in about 7 percent of my patients, slightly less frequently than carpal tunnel syndrome. With appropriate ergonomic intervention, coupled with rest and physical therapy for radial tunnel syndrome, results are good.

Some surgeons propose surgery if there is no improvement after four months of conservative treatment to forestall permanent nerve damage. As with all surgery, it should be considered a last resort. About 30 percent of the time, tennis elbow and radial tunnel syndrome occur simultaneously, leading some health professionals to call it resistant tennis elbow. However, when radial tunnel syndrome occurs alone, it can be mistaken for tennis elbow. Only clinical evaluation can clear this up.

Cervical Nerve Root Compression

Also known as cervical radiculopathy, this is sometimes over-diagnosed as a cause of pain and other symptoms in RSI. There is a definite tendency to underdiagnose neurogenic thoracic outlet syndrome. I have found cervical radiculopathy in only 0.03 percent of my patients, although this low number may not hold for a population older than my patients, who had a mean age of 38.5 years. A focused physical exam will usually make the distinction. Cervical radiculopathy usually involves the C5-C7 disc area in the neck. In cervical nerve root compression, weakness occurs in muscle groups such as the deltoids, the serratus, rotator cuff, and biceps. In neurogenic thoracic outlet syndrome (TOS), which usually involves the C7-C8-T1 area of the spine, weakness occurs in the hand and forearm muscles. Another distinction is that there is a tendency to drop things in TOS because of weakness in the hand and forearm muscles.

In adulthood, many of us have protruding discs, which may lead to a diagnosis of root compression when seen on X-ray. A complete exam and certain specific tests such as MRIs and nerve conduction studies may be necessary if there is any doubt. It should not be forgotten that cervical discs and neurogenic thoracic outlet could occur simultaneously. Thus, cervical radiculopathy can occur from acute or chronic hernia of a disc. A disc is a cushion of cartilage between vertebrae and can be associated with the slipping of one vertebra over another (spondylolisthesis) or a bony proliferation occluding the hole (foramen) from which the spinal nerve exits. Tumors of the cervical cord can also cause symptoms of radiculopathy. A major complaint is pain, first in the neck followed by shoulder, forearm, and hand; the pain can be made worse by exaggerated neck movements, including whiplash. Diagnosis is made by X-rays, EMGs, CT scans, MRIs of the spine, and other lab tests and by observing for motor weakness and diminished deep tendon reflexes. A C5–C6 disc lesion produces weakness of the biceps, and a C6–C7 disc lesion produces weakness of the triceps and deltoids.

Clinical diagnosis requires a Spurling's test, where the head is tilted toward the involved side and pressure is applied to the top of the head, eliciting pain. If there is a history of whiplash injury or other injury suggestive of cervical root compression, consultation with a neurologist or neurosurgeon should be sought.

Any manipulation or treatment of the neck before ruling out cervical radiculopathy might cause serious injury.

Injury to Tendons

Tendons are attached on either end of muscles and transmit mechanical movement of the muscles to the bone. Tendons are dynamic structures with a rich supply of nerves, permitting them to perceive the degree of tension (proprioception), which is transmitted back to the brain or the spinal column. Tendons also have specific blood supplies, which can vary in different areas of the tendons. Because tendons are generally smaller in the upper extremities, they are particularly at risk for inflammation (tendinitis). With injury, the exquisitely regular microscopic architecture of the tendon becomes disorganized and is repaired with scar tissue, which permanently shortens the tendon. When a tendon tears or is acutely injured, minimal splinting during treatment to allow some motion of the tendon during healing will keep the scarring to a minimum. Tendons perform a variety of functions. One is that they allow several muscles to act on one site. When tendons become inflamed or irritated and swollen from repetitive movement through a constricting sheath, you have a condition called tenosynovitis. Outlined below are some of the more common forms of tendon injury that we see in people with RSI.

Medial epicondylitis (golfer's elbow), which I have found in more than 60 percent of my patients with RSI, is the most frequent form of tendinitis. Lateral epicondylitis (tennis elbow), at more than 30 percent, is less common than medial epicondylitis in people with RSI.

In DeQuervain's tenosynovitis we are dealing with a slightly different mechanism of injury (see figure 9). In this case the tendons are attached to the muscles that move the thumb in an upward and outward direction. Because the tendons change direction as they move they can become injured by friction in the sheath and become inflamed.

People who develop DeQuervain's—18 percent of my patients—usually engage in biomechanically harmful positioning of the thumb. Often they raise their thumbs above the space bar of the keyboard to keep the space bar free for the other thumb, or they grip the mouse too tightly. Pianists who cross their thumb far into the palm while doing scales or arpeggios; violinists who grip the neck of the violin tightly to keep it from sliding off their shoulders; or clarinetists whose right thumb supports are too low, are all candidates for DeQuervain's.*

Flexor tendinitis, or trigger finger, is another common ailment in RSI. The hand has no muscles from the knuckle joint (metacarpal joint) to the tip of the finger. The mechanism for moving the fingers relies primarily on muscles in the forearm attached to long tendons, which form a set of pulleys in the fingers. Inflammation of these tendons and their sheaths hinders free movement of the wrist and fingers and is associated with stiffness, pain, and loss of range of motion. Awkward positioning and tight gripping can contribute to the development of this condition, which also can lead to trigger finger.

---

*An article in the *New York Times* of April 30, 2002, titled "Youth Let Their Thumbs Do the Talking in Japan," notes an interesting phenomenon. Japanese youngsters are increasingly using Web-capable phones that require the use of both thumbs to push their buttons. Television stations in Japan have even held thumb-speed contests, with one woman clocked at a hundred Chinese characters per minute, the equivalent of a touch-typing speed of a hundred words per minute. The ultimate effect of this in leading to injury such as DeQuervain's tenosynovitis remains to be seen.

Many of my RSI patients had evidence of shoulder range of motion impairment, which is related to postural misalignment. The shoulder is the most mobile joint in the body. The ball of the upper arm bone (humerus) is not enclosed in a deep cup, like the hip joint. Instead, the upper arm bone rests in a shallow cup surrounded by a circle of muscles, ligaments, and tendons that stabilize it and work the joint (the rotator cuff). Tightening and contraction of these muscles can lead to restriction of shoulder motion. Carried a step farther, this tightening can result in the head of the humerus being pulled up against the bones of the scapula and clavicle, resulting in what is called shoulder impingement. This restricted shoulder movement becomes painful when extreme movements are attempted. A frozen shoulder occurs when most shoulder movement becomes impossible. Degenerated muscles and tendons of the rotator cuff can easily tear either partially or completely during lifting movements or a fall, causing severe pain. Tears need immediate attention and possibly surgery.

Correcting these conditions is critical because performing activities with limited shoulder movement shifts the workload to the more delicate forearm and hand muscles. I have found impaired shoulder range of motion in more than 40 percent of my patients and shoulder impingement in more than 10 percent.

Bicipital tendinitis occurs when the tendons of the biceps muscle become irritated in a groove at the shoulder. Postural misalignment is usually associated with this condition. I found that 15 percent of my patients had evidence of bicipital tendinitis.

Injury to Muscles

Muscles are the engines that drive all of the movements in the body. For muscles to do their job, they must be well supplied with nutrients and must be connected to functioning nerves. Muscles that are not in balance with other muscles can instigate events that can cause damage to all soft tissues. Earlier, we reviewed the cascading factors in postural deterioration where a conflict between muscle groups damages nerves and other soft tissues and, ultimately, many other muscles of the body.

Oddly, little emphasis has been placed on the important role of muscles in RSI. The lack of sufficient healthy muscle to carry out life's functions is ultimately the distinguishing characteristic of RSI. RSI sufferers have weakness, soreness, and tenderness in compromised muscles, and as the illness progresses, the muscles contract, leading to nerve compression or traction, loss of normal joint range of motion, and the entire spectrum of RSI disabilities.

Muscles are highly complex, sensitive structures that have exquisite capabilities to adapt to a variety of uses. Lift weights to gain strength, and old muscle fibers will be broken down and replaced with new fibers, more capable of sustaining increased loading. This phenomenon is known as the degeneration/regeneration cycle. For muscle to regenerate normally, nerve stimulus, an adequate supply of the stem cells called satellite cells, good blood supply, and certain hormones are necessary. If one or more of these factors is lacking, muscle regeneration will be thwarted.

The way in which muscles are used can accelerate injury. Consider the person with RSI whose posture has caused nerve dysfunction and who with repetitive motion is therefore tearing down muscle fibers at a prodigious rate but who now has limited capacity to regenerate new muscle. This is something we often see in people who use their bodies in a biomechanically poor fashion, increasing the likelihood of injury. The more of this kind of malpositioning, the more potential for injury. This type of muscle activity leads to disruption of the muscle's calcium metabolism and produces disorganization of muscle structure.

When muscles are injured they release chemicals that stimulate the nerve fibers, causing pain. Palpation of muscles in the hands, forearms, neck, and upper back reveals soreness and contraction. With more severe injury, swelling and inflammation occur.

These manifestations of muscle injury are sometimes called myofascial pain syndrome, implying that not only muscle but also its surrounding cover (fascia) have sustained injury. I have found some form of myofascial pain syndrome extremely common in RSI and it was found in most of my patients.

Fibromyalgia

The term fibromyalgia, now part of the medical lexicon, is difficult to define and is surrounded by controversy. Most of the time there seems to be no cause for the condition, though it has sometimes been linked to surgery or trauma. Janet Travell, who became famous as John F. Kennedy's physician, identified a series of trigger points or tender areas that cause pain when pressure is applied. Symptoms of fibromyalgia include muscle stiffness and pain, fatigue, headaches, abdominal distension, diarrhea, and bladder irritation. The American College of Rheumatology has endorsed diagnostic criteria relating to eighteen painful points where muscle, tendon, and ligament attach to bone. If eleven of these painful points are noted, especially when accompanied by other symptoms, a patient is said to have fibromyalgia.

Since these points are located where tendons insert into bone, they are probably related to muscle tightness and imbalance. Causes may include mental or physical stress as well as anxiety and depression. Fibromyalgia is reported most frequently in women. Treatment is no different from what I propose for RSI: a team approach with physical or occupational therapy, a home exercise program, psychological counseling, and use of medications where indicated.

Injury to Ligaments

The term ligament implies a tying together, and indeed ligaments tie muscle to bone. But ligaments are also dynamic structures that play an active role in maintaining joint stability and sending signals to the brain regarding their status (proprioception). Ligaments control the limits of joint movements, prohibiting exaggerated actions. In the early stages of child development, ligaments undergo tissue modification to become spinal discs and joint surfaces.

Loose ligaments can destabilize joints. For example, loose ligaments create greater risk of injury by making it more difficult
for "double-jointed" people to maintain a stable hand. I have
noted a high incidence of hyperlaxity of finger and elbow joints,
especially in women. In certain fingers and in the elbows, the
incidence is well over 50 percent. People with RSI who are
hyperlax need biomechanical retraining to teach appropriate
positioning of the hand and the fingers, so as to create a more stable arch of the fingers. Long fingernails will make this impossible; they must be cut to a length no greater than one-sixteenth of
an inch. People with hyperlaxity of the elbows and other joints
must be careful not to overstretch these joints when exercising.

Ganglions

If you develop a lump or a bump in the hand, it is probably a
ganglion cyst. These are soft-tissue "blowouts," which can occur
on the tendon, the tendon sheaths, or the cells lining the joint.
They look like a round bump under the skin. Most of the time
they do not produce symptoms, but sometimes they can put
pressure on nerves, especially in the Guyon's canal or the cubital
tunnel, where they cause nerve compression. The top or dorsum
of the wrist is where I have most commonly found ganglion cysts

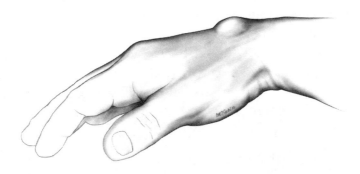

Figure 16. A ganglion cyst is a common location for these tendon-related soft-tissue
"blowouts."

(about 13 percent). There is no harm in leaving them, unless they are compressing a nerve or an artery.

Linburg's Tendon Anomaly

Because I have found Linburg's tendon anomaly in 13 percent of the people I have examined, I believe this is worth noting. Linburg's tendon is an extra slip of tendon connecting a flexor tendon of the thumb to a flexor tendon of the index finger. When you pull the thumb toward your palm, it causes curling of the tip of the index finger. Conversely, if you grasp the tip of the index finger, it can prevent the thumb from moving toward the palm. This condition can sometimes cause problems in finger action for computer users or musicians. Biomechanical rehabilitation can prevent the problems associated with this anomaly.

TFCC Tears

If a patient with RSI complains of pain in the ulnar portion of the wrist, I consider the possibility of a perforation or tear of the stabilizing wrist structure at the joint between the radius and the ulna bones. This is called the triangular fibrocartilaginous complex (TFCC). A TFCC tear can occur in people who have had a previous wrist fracture or a traumatic wrist dislocation. It can also result from excessive frequent movement, from pronation to supination. Pain in the ulnar portion of the wrist is a frequent complaint. Although computer use or other repetitive tasks do not usually cause a TFCC tear, it affects the quality of work and should be considered in a patient history. Diagnosis is confirmed by MRI. Treatment, which should be undertaken by a hand specialist, will vary based on the character of the lesion.

Other Injuries

While not directly related to RSI, the ligament of the thumb known as the ulnar collateral ligament can sustain a tear, particularly among people with joint hyperlaxity. Ulnar collateral ligament tear is sometimes called gamekeeper's thumb, because it was first described in gamekeepers, whose work included twisting the necks of small game. It commonly occurs from a fall on an outstretched hand or in a fall with the strap of a ski pole in the hand. This tear can be disabling because it causes instability of the thumb while typing or gripping a mouse. If the disability is severe, surgery may be indicated.

Pain caused by the superficial branch of the radial nerve, or Wartenburg's syndrome, is rare—I've seen it in only three of almost five hundred patients, twice in relation to tight splints used to treat carpal tunnel syndrome. Occasionally the superficial branch of the radial nerve can be compressed, giving rise to numbness, burning pain, and night pain along the back of the wrist, in the thumb, and in the web space between the thumb and index finger. Even the touch of clothing in this region can produce tingling. In another case, a tight wristwatch band was the cause. This injury to the radial nerve has been reported as a complication of the surgery for DeQuervain's disease.

Thrombophlebitis in Computer Users: "Economy Class Syndrome"

A potential threat to computer users who spend long hours seated at a desk is the possibility that they will develop thrombophlebitis, or blood clots in the veins of the legs. This is similar to what has been reported in airline passengers who take long flights in cramped economy class seats. Although considered rare in computer users, it may be more common than previously thought. Both Richard Nixon and Dan Quayle—hardly typical economy class fliers—developed this illness.

Ordinarily, sitting for a long time may cause small clots to develop that gradually dissipate after you get up and move around. An extreme example was reported by a group of physicians from New Zealand who wrote about a thirty-two-year-old man who spent up to twelve hours daily at his workstation, hardly ever getting up. He began to notice swelling in his calves followed about ten days later with shortness of breath, a sign that some clots had broken off and migrated to his lungs. He soon became unconscious, and was hospitalized. Tests confirmed the clots in his lungs. He survived, but needed more than six months of treatment with anticlotting medications. Other physicians have reported seeing people with similar symptoms. A London physician speaking recently to reporters at Reuters Health Information says we may be seeing more of this illness, especially if we look for it during examination. It should be stressed, however, that this complication may be relatively rare. To avoid thrombophlebitis, computer users should take a break every hour, get up, walk around, and do some basic foot and leg exercises. Taking hourly breaks will also benefit vision and general muscle function. Computer users should note that coexisting illnesses such as diabetes or a heart condition might increase the risk of "economy class syndrome."

Getting the Diagnosis Right

Unusual symptoms can present a serious challenge to the evaluating physician. One of my patients, B. Z., was a thirty-five-year-old woman whose work involved about six hours daily at a computer, most of it combined with speaking to clients on the telephone. Apart from an auto accident two years previously, which resulted in a whiplash injury, B. Z. was in good health. The neck pain from the whiplash resolved in a few days and did not bother her subsequently. Her troubles began when she decided to paint her bedroom by herself. She spent several hours with a brush in her right hand while holding the paint can for part of the time in her left hand. The following day she noticed the onset of a headache on her left side. The pain was piercing and over the next few days got worse, extending over her eye and on the left side of her face and neck. It was accompanied by numbness and tingling. Over time the symptoms migrated down her left arm. After about a week the headache was so severe that she was unable to work. Acetaminophen and NSAIDs gave little or no relief. B. Z. sought help in her local emergency department, and after a perfunctory exam, an ER physician gave her some commonly used preparations for migraine headache. Despite the medication, her headache persisted. She then sought the help of her HMO plan's primary care physician, who after hearing her symptoms called a colleague neurologist who said that her symptoms "didn't make any sense" and that she was probably a hysteric, a label often directed at women when the diagnosis is not textbook-clear. As her symptoms persisted, she saw the chief neurologist at her HMO. As she had not lost strength in her upper body function to any great degree, he ruled out a stroke and sent her for an MRI, suspecting multiple sclerosis. But the MRI and other tests were negative, and he told her "it was probably in her head" (which it was!) and gave her no further appointments. She was still in considerable distress when we saw her. The clinical tests for neurogenic thoracic outlet syndrome, none of which had been performed by any of her physicians, were dramatically positive on her left side, and she was long-necked with drooping shoulders, which are risk factors for neurogenic TOS. After several weeks of physical therapy and home exercises her symptoms abated, but even when symptom-free, when she did overhead chores she noted a "strange feeling," which would go away if she did more intensive stretching.

This case illustrates several issues. First, the need for a complete physical exam in such cases; second, the need for even specialists to rely on their clinical expertise when performing these exams; third, the importance of obtaining a thorough history—in this case, the whiplash injury might have set the stage for the later injury; fourth, the need for health professionals to know about the link between neurogenic thoracic outlet syndrome and migrainelike headaches; and fifth, the responsibility of the health professional to avoid accusations of "hysteria" before ruling out every possible physical cause for unpleasant symptoms.

The lesson: RSI and its complications can often be mistaken for emotional or neurological disease. If the cause of the symptoms is not obvious to the examiner it can easily be sorted out by a methodical clinical approach and some basic clinical tests. RSI is a very complex illness with many possible findings, which can usually be discerned through a thorough physical evaluation. These findings are the bases for diagnosis, which establishes the rationale for a focused, team-oriented treatment program. Though a complete upper-body physical may reveal some of these conditions, periodic general examinations should be part of your normal health regimen.

The case of Mr. C, a fifty-year-old manager in a small electronics company, illustrates the complexities of the physical examination of a patient with upper-extremity symptoms. Mr. C's work entails a good deal of stressful customer relations, about two to four hours of computer work, and about two hours a day of driving. He is a nonsmoker who has been in generally good health. Eleven years prior to his visit he noted some neck pain and shoulder discomfort, which led him to see a chiropractor. While undergoing a manipulation on his neck, Mr. C felt a sudden "popping" accompanied by severe and sudden pain. X-rays and CT scans of the neck revealed that a ruptured disc was protruding and compressing his spinal column at the C5–C6 level. He suddenly lost the normal curvature of his cervical spine due to muscle spasm. A week after this occurrence, Mr. C underwent discectomy, the surgical removal of the rubbery disc between adjacent bony vertebrae. The two adjacent segments were fused as part of the operation, resulting in the loss of flexibility between the C5 and C6 vertebrae. Cervical degenerative disc disease is about a fifth as common as low back disc problems. The C5–C6 level in the neck is where this most commonly occurs.

Mr. C may not have been given a sufficient period of conservative management before resorting to surgery. Conservative management would have included a neck brace, rest, pain medication, and focused physical therapy including home exercises and possibly psychological intervention. It might not have worked for Mr. C, but probably it should have been the initial approach. Following this surgical intervention, pain diminished but did not disappear. This residual pain was described as "different." Several months later, an evaluation revealed the presence of another protruding disc at the C6–C7 level. This time conservative treatment was followed. Physical therapy exercises were prescribed and were helpful. Over several years Mr. C experienced increasing pain affecting the upper extremities. Gradually his activities became more restricted. He could no longer drive comfortably, and he gave up gardening and most sports, but he continued to work. He restricted his office work to three days a week to minimize his driving. As his life became more restricted he saw a number of physicians who recommended a variety of treatment approaches while always assuming his symptoms were from his disc-related cervical radiculopathy. His pain then took on a burning quality, particularly in the lower neck area and shoulders along the upper trapezius muscle. It was more severe on the left. This seemed to suggest that his sympathetic nervous system was now involved. Soon afterward he began to notice that his hands were getting colder, and he began to drop things from his left hand. Low back pain also ensued due to a compensatory imbalance of the spine, since the entire spine works in a synchronous fashion. He was given a variety of medications to control his symptoms, including a gastroprotective NSAID, a muscle relaxant, and antidepressant medications, including both an SSRI and a tricyclic (see chapter 5). Despite these measures, his condition worsened.

At this juncture an evaluating physician should look for new causes of the symptoms, since many of the new complaints were not compatible with disc disease alone. Physical examination revealed a host of new findings, including clinical signs of neurogenic thoracic outlet syndrome, reflex sympathetic dysfunction, myofascial pain syndrome, golfer's elbow, shoulder weakness, and depression. The results of the physical exam pointed to a mixed syndrome of a more complex nature, which would make treatment more difficult. One example of this difficulty would be the treatment of Mr. C's lack of neck range of motion, which helped to cause the nerve traction and compression of the brachial plexus. The therapist would be loath to force the neck into various positions for fear of further damage to the spine. Instead, soft tissue work would have to be applied to stretch the neck muscles passively. Next, the weakness of the shoulders, arms, forearms, and hand would need to be addressed with stretching and strengthening where indicated. A carefully choreographed home exercise program could then be started.

Mr. C's condition did improve with this approach, but it took almost a year of intense therapy. He was finally able to drive comfortably. He made appropriate ergonomic changes in his workstation and was careful about pacing himself. Mr. C's experience demonstrates the need to recognize that many factors are at play in those who present with work-related upper-body disorders. They often pose diagnostic challenges that can only be solved by a methodical physical exam followed by aggressive and focused intervention.

3

RSI and Your Emotions

There can be no transforming of darkness into light and
of apathy into movement without emotion.

—Carl Jung, 1875–1961

Repetitive strain injury is often associated with disabling emotional and psychological problems. Stress, chronic pain, complex chronic pain, anxiety, depression, and panic are all linked and can lead to a fearsome chain of events that needs to be broken before it causes or increases disability.

While most of the emotional and psychological problems we see result from RSI and the damage it causes, they also can be a contributing cause of RSI in the first place. Typically, while under minimal stress, you might be working long hours at an ergonomically poor workstation with awkward posture and positioning, when pain and other RSI symptoms develop. In this case, stress follows increasing pain, which then leads to anxiety. As the pain and discomfort become more difficult to control, severe emotional problems can develop.

Conversely, someone working long hours in a stressful environment, perhaps having problems with an employer or fellow employee, may become stressed and tense. With increasing stress levels, muscles can become tight, pain follows, muscle injury increases as work continues, and the harmful cycle has begun.

Surviving the emotional and physical roller coaster of RSI requires help from professionals who are familiar with this disabling combination. Rarely can you rise above the physical problems of RSI without having to deal with the emotional component as well.

Stress

Stress is your body's reaction to any disturbing physical, mental, or emotional stimulus. In 1953, Hans Selye described stress as a basic defense mechanism characterized by fight or flight. Adrenaline levels rise and in turn stimulate the body to secrete hormones to prepare it for an encounter. Dr. Selye described two kinds of stress: eustress (good stress) and distress (bad stress). Stress is not always harmful. Eustress is beneficial to the body and can result from moderate physical exercise—the pleasant rush you feel after a vigorous workout. Distress is the extreme form of stress. Some examples of distress are excessive exercise, overwork, or lack of sleep. Distress is likely to lead to anxiety and depression and in severe instances to panic reactions.

Anxiety Disorders

Anxiety can be heightened by fear about the cause and outcome of your illness. The best way to begin coping with your anxiety is to seek a complete evaluation by a knowledgeable physician who will discuss your problem in depth and put it in perspective for you. Understanding RSI can be very reassuring and will enable you to take charge of your situation and begin changing things.

A common fear in RSI is that you can lose your job, your means of sustenance, and your health. Understanding that there is a process that you can go through to preserve your health will help you deal with the realistic worry and anger you may feel about these overwhelming occurrences.

Anxiety can involve a variety of circumstances, including fears of social situations such as public speaking, physical environmental fears such as crowds or cramped spaces, and trauma such as the soft-tissue injury encountered in RSI or an auto accident. As if in double jeopardy, the RSI patient is at risk for the effects of job loss or the threat of job loss. Separation or death of a family member or friend can also contribute to anxiety.

Anxiety disorders have been classified by the American Psychiatric Association so that they can be better understood and treated. The classification for anxiety disorders includes the following:

- adjustment disorder with anxious features

- acute stress disorder

- generalized anxiety disorder

- phobic disorders, including specific phobia, social phobia, and agoraphobia

- post-traumatic stress disorder

- panic disorder

- obsessive-compulsive disorder

With RSI, we are most likely to encounter three of these: generalized anxiety disorder (GAD), post-traumatic stress disorder (PTSD), and panic disorder.

If anxiety symptoms come on suddenly, it is important to perform a medical evaluation, which should include tests for thyroid and pulmonary diseases such as asthma or COPD. Drugs that can be misused or overused that can lead to anxiety include caffeine, cocaine, methamphetamines, thyroid medications, or bronchodilators used for asthma. Alcohol or benzodiazepines, particularly if they are discontinued abruptly, can result in acute anxiety.

Research suggests that the part of the brain that may play a role as a mediator for anxiety is the amygdala, an almond-shaped mass of gray matter located in the front part of the temporal lobe of the brain.

Generalized Anxiety Disorder (GAD)

The association of GAD with RSI is probably more common than realized. It is also worth noting that many of the symptoms of GAD are also found in reflex sympathetic dysfunction, which can occur in almost 20 percent of RSI patients. In both conditions there is increased sympathetic nervous system outflow, producing cold, clammy hands, sweating, muscle tension, trembling, twitching, aching, and soreness. Dry mouth, nausea, diarrhea, and urinary frequency are also common.

GAD is characterized by a long-term siege of worry that is difficult to control and anxiety symptoms such as restlessness, easy fatigability, irritability, sleep problems, and muscle tension. The diagnosis of GAD is made by a psychiatrist, but the intervention of a medical specialist is also a wise idea, since a medical condition such as alcoholism or drug abuse needs to be ruled out.

Treatment should be supervised by a psychiatrist, who may decide to make follow-up referrals to various therapeutic groups. The inciting cause, such as job loss or injury from a repetitive motion injury, also needs to be remedied. There are many medications considered effective for GAD. These include benzodiazepines; tricyclic antidepressants; buspirone, a nonaddicting antianxiety agent; selective serotonin uptake inhibitors (SSRIs); trazadone; and venlafaxine antidepressants. These medications should be administered strictly under the supervision of a psychiatrist.

Post-traumatic Stress Disorder (PTSD)

Soft-tissue injury encountered in RSI might lead to post-traumatic stress disorder, which was studied extensively in Vietnam veterans. It is being increasingly recognized as a result of many types of injury. The characteristics of PTSD include traumatic exposure when a person experiences, witnesses, or is confronted with events that involve serious injury, threatened death, or a threat to the physical integrity of oneself or others. The person with PTSD experiences an intense fear accompanied by a feeling of helplessness or horror. Many patients I have seen who are confronted with repetitive strain injury, combined with loss of job or difficulties at work, fit this description.

PTSD is now recognized as a fairly common disorder, with a lifetime prevalence as high as 8 percent. Women are affected twice as often as men. As in RSI, once exposed, there is an increased risk for another episode. Symptoms of PTSD can include nightmares, flashbacks, emotional numbness, and trouble concentrating. The most effective medications for PTSD are SSRI antidepressants administered under the care of a psychiatrist who has made the diagnosis.

Panic Disorder

The emotional components related to job loss and stress can lead to panic disorder. These can occur as unexpected attacks consisting of acute paroxysms of anxiety. A physician making the diagnosis would note shortness of breath, rapid heart rate, light-headedness, sweating, tremor. and nausea. Panic disorder can even mimic a heart attack. Also characteristic of a panic disorder is a definite feeling of fear and a desire to flee. Women have a greater propensity to develop it than men, and it generally occurs in the late teens through the thirties. It can be accompanied by agoraphobia, major depression, substance abuse, and risk of suicide. This can adversely affect quality of life. As with other anxiety disorders, panic reaction is often unrecognized by medical doctors.

After diagnosis the managing physician can choose from a variety of medications added to psychiatric counseling. These include the benzodiazepines; monoamine oxidase inhibitors; SSRIs; tricyclic antidepressants; and venlafaxine, which is an antidepressant unrelated to other groups.

Depression

The depression associated with RSI is generally considered a transient and reactive mood disorder that subsides when the injury heals. This type of depression is a response to a complex set of disturbing circumstances such as soft-tissue injury, loss of self-esteem, job insecurity, financial problems, or strained relationships with an employer, fellow employees, or family. Even athletes who suffer an injury in their sport may find themselves in depression, which subsides after the healing of their injury. Depression can be part of the comorbidity picture described with certain anxiety disorders.

If you are depressed, a stimulant is not the appropriate medication. Depression and stimulants are a dangerous combination that can lead to paranoid suicidal thinking. Seek help if there are any signs of depressive behavior.

The incidence of emotional and mental disturbances is high in people with RSI. A psychiatrist or psychologist can be helpful. Anyone with previous mental health problems may have a recurrence with RSI. There are antidepressant medications that are useful in controlling the depression as well as the pain of RSI. They are discussed in chapter 5.

The first sign of work-related emotional upheaval would be a good time to get your problem diagnosed and a treatment program begun. Begin with an emotional assessment as well as a physical or occupational therapy assessment. Then make sure you have corrected any ergonomic deficiencies at work and that you pace yourself by taking adequate rest breaks, which will relieve some stress.

The emotional problems that accompany RSI don't go away easily, and you may need to have psychiatric or psychological counseling. Initially it is probably wise to seek the individual counseling of a psychiatrist or psychologist. This is important, because professional expertise is necessary to rule out any serious problems that need continuing care. Another important reason to seek the help of a mental health professional is the possibility that you might benefit from the use of antidepressants or other medications. These medications also might increase your tolerance to pain by raising your pain threshold and making it easier for you to participate in physical therapy and exercise.

In a professionally run support group conducted by a psychotherapist or social worker, you can find a safe haven where you can discuss your problem. The professionals will be able to determine if there is anyone with a severe emotional problem requiring medication or a more sophisticated level of care.

There are many peer-run RSI support groups, usually in major cities. Participating in a group affiliated with your workplace is one option, though the privacy of such a group may be limited.

Information about how to find these groups is in the Internet resources section.

4

RSI and Your
Eyes

Don't go looking at me like that, because you'll wear your
eyes out.

–Émile Zola, *La Bête Humaine*

If you have had any problems with headaches, blurred vision, or
eyestrain, this chapter will help you understand what is happening and help you discuss your eye condition more easily with
your doctor. Like any fine and complex instrument, eyes need
to be cared for and allowed to do their job under the best conditions possible. It is important that any computer user with eye
problems see an eye specialist such as an ophthalmologist. When
you begin sustained work at the computer, you may notice that
your day-to-day corrective lenses won't work as well for you, and
a new lens prescription just for computer work may be necessary.

Eye Checkups

Our eyes were not designed for the strains of office work. As a
result, every year millions of people consult eye specialists for
problems that begin with computer use. As early as 1977, a

Swedish study conducted on airline reservation clerks, showed that 75 percent of them complained of vision problems, while 55 percent had shoulder and back pain and 35 percent suffered with headaches and neck stiffness. Is this still the case for present-day computer users? The answer appears to be yes. James Sheedy, O.D., Ph.D., who is now director of professional development at Sola Optical USA, has reported that 75 percent of all computer users suffer from a variety of eyesight-related problems, which he ranks in order of frequency:

- eyestrain

- headache

- blurred vision

- temporary myopia (nearsightedness)

- dry or irritated eyes

- neck and backache

- photophobia (sensitivity to light)

- double vision

- afterimages

If you have any of these problems, seek the help necessary to remedy it. Each of these conditions can probably be corrected by proper intervention.

Computer Vision Syndrome

Eye problems relating to the use of the computer are sometimes called computer vision syndrome (CVS). It is said that 60 million people suffer from these eye problems and that the number is rising by 1 million yearly. Your eyes perform an enormous amount of work when you use your computer. CVS exists partly because the image on the CRT computer screen is constantly being reprojected at a rapid frequency (the refresh rate). (This is not the case with an LCD or plasma monitor.) Print on paper is more distinct than the images you see on the computer

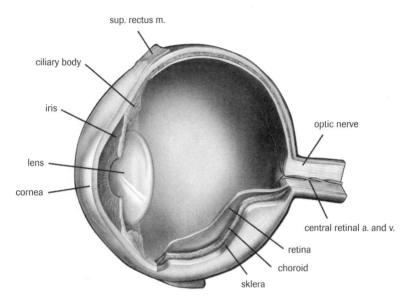

Figure 17. Side view of the eye. Attached internal muscles adjust the lens to change focus.

monitor, which are created by red, green, and blue dots that continually flash on the screen too rapidly for you to detect. So the refresh rate is far from refreshing. Some other causes of CVS include long hours at the computer, poor ergonomic setups, and poor vision correction.

The eye is a complex organ capable of many functions, a number of which have important bearings on vision at the workstation. One of these functions is called accommodation. The closest distance that allows you to focus sharply on an object is called the near point of accommodation. Internal eye muscles adjust the lens to make focusing possible. As we age, lens elasticity diminishes, causing the near point to move farther away. This is why at about forty years of age, many of us need bifocals.

You can improve your accommodation by looking down slightly. If you look up or sideways, the ability to accommodate diminishes. Therefore, when looking at your computer monitor, depending on the distance your eyes are from the screen (normally arm's length), you should be viewing the center of the

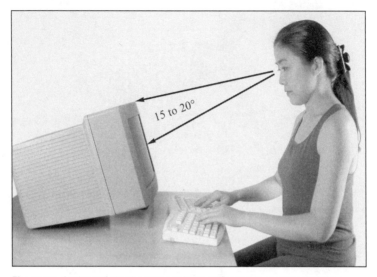

Figure 18. Acuity and visual acuity can improve by setting up your monitor so that you look down at it.

monitor screen at a downward angle. As you see from the illustration on this page, a straight line from the top of the monitor to the level of your eyes should result in a 15- to 20-degree downward angle to the center of the screen.

As you get nearer to the screen, a greater downward angle will be necessary to focus clearly, so avoid neck and back strain by staying as near arm's length as possible. When you gaze downward at the computer, bend from the hips, not just the neck. A slight chin tuck can relieve neck strain when looking down.

Another important function is binocularity, which is the ability of our eyes to fuse the images from each eye into a single, three-dimensional image. If this function is disturbed and the image in each eye is seen at different levels, it is called heterophoria, a fairly common condition that is often ignored. Attempts to compensate for heterophoria can cause tilting of the head and neck or other awkward postures, resulting in both neck pain and eyestrain. Your ophthalmologist usually can correct or improve heterophoria.

Another important but often neglected factor is the determination of your eye dominance. You may not be aware of it, but you probably favor one eye over the other, just as you may be right-handed or left-handed. Right-handedness doesn't always coincide with right-eye dominance. About 40 percent of people are "crossovers"–their eye dominance is the opposite of their hand dominance. Knowing your eye dominance can help you adjust your workstation more efficiently. A right-handed person who is left-eye-dominant, yet places the bulk of documents used in his work on the right, will be turning his or her head sharply to the right to bring the left eye into focusing position. If, instead, the documents are placed on the left, he or she will do less head turning. With some kinds of computer work such as data entry, the user may be more comfortable with the data placed more centrally and the monitor moved slightly closer toward the dominant eye. Alternatively, a document holder on the dominant eye side may be more comfortable. If you offset the screen slightly from center to favor your dominant eye you may feel more comfortable, although LCD screens may become more difficult to see.

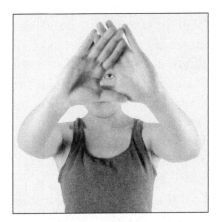

Figure 19. It's easy to figure out your eye dominance. Form a small hole between your index fingers and your thumbs, with arms fully extended. Look at a single object through the hole formed by your hands and draw your hands toward your face while keeping your eyes on the object. The hole made by your hands will be in front of your dominant eye.

Choosing the Right Visual Tools

Your goal is to achieve visual comfort and visual safety. Choices should be made with the help of an ophthalmologist or other qualified vision specialist.

Not everyone will need the same type of correction for computer use. For people with 20/20 vision or better, no intervention may be required. People who wear lenses have several options. For near- or farsightedness, with or without astigmatism, simple refraction may be all that is necessary. Those over forty, who need bifocals because their near point of visual acuity has lengthened, have several options: ordinary bifocals, progressive lenses, special computer screen lenses, contact lenses, screen lenses that enlarge the screen image, LCD projection, or an LCD or plasma screen.

Ordinary bifocals can cause neck and back problems because they force you to tilt your head back to see the screen clearly. If you are not a touch typist, you will be in an awkward viewing position when you look at the keyboard.

Progressive lenses may be slightly better than traditional bifocals, but like traditional bifocals, may restrict side vision, so that you may not see the full width of the monitor and adjacent reading materials. A new type of lens created especially for the computer user, the Continuum lens, claims to allow the bifocal user to see the entire workspace more comfortably.

Bifocal contact lenses may offer a slightly greater visual field than ordinary bifocals. Contact lens users tend to get dry eyes. Low humidity can contribute to dry eyes, too. Blinking more frequently can help, as can artificial tears without vasoconstrictors. Blinking reminder programs are available for the computer.

Screen lenses are another visual tool involving the application of a special lens in front of the screen. One type is called the PC Magni-viewer. However, a larger PC screen can do as well as a screen lens.

LCD projection or large LCD or plasma screens are tools that can be used for serious visual deficiencies. See the visual aids section, which follows.

Using only dark letters on a light background can aid eye comfort. Rest your eyes for several minutes of each workhour by looking away from the screen or by gazing at distant objects. Keep your lenses and your monitor screen clean.

To achieve a visually ergonomic workstation, a computer user should pay attention to positioning, angling his or her monitor correctly, controlling glare, distortion, reflection and flicker as well as modifying work lighting if necessary.

Start by having your screen straight up and down (at a right angle to the desk). The screen is then gradually tilted upward, toward your face, until it feels comfortable and you see clearly. Studies have shown that there is greater comfort and less visual distortion with this approach, but the upward-facing screen can produce glare by catching ceiling lights.

There are several ways by which lighting problems can be solved. Turn off your screen and look for reflection and light sources. Decrease overhead lighting by using a hood for the screen, something that can be purchased or fashioned out of cardboard. Reduce glare by directing the monitor screen away from windows and light sources. Use glare screens if necessary— these are available at computer stores. Indirect lighting aimed away from the workstation can diffuse light and diminish reflection. If you can see flickering on your screen, lower the brightness of the monitor.

Each computer job presents its own challenges to eye comfort at the workstation. These job characteristics were classified by Professor Étienne Grandjean and updated by Stuart B. Leavitt, Ph.D., C.I.E., of Leavitt Communications.

Here are some tips that may help you at your workstation:

Data document entry. The main job here is to read documents and enter data into the computer system. In this kind of work, the keyboard and screen are secondary to the document being read. Locate your reference documents centrally, and keep the monitor slightly on the side of your dominant eye.

Data search/inquiry with data insertion. The Internet user, transcriptionist, and telemarketer all work at the computer in this manner. Here, attention is directed primarily at the screen. A telephone is often an additional data source. Keep the monitor in front of you or slightly to the side of your dominant eye, and make sure the monitor and keyboard are at comfortable angles. If you work with a phone at your computer, get a headset.

Interactive use. Travel reservationists and banking personnel, for example, are involved in data entry and data acquisition at the computer and also must have access to printed documents. Try to align your documents toward the side of your dominant eye; a document holder attached to the side of the monitor case is useful here.

Design and graphics. Computer-aided design (CAD), computer-aided manufacturing (CAM), and desktop publishing (DTP) are usually done with pointing devices like the mouse or puck and a large-screen monitor. Here the keyboard is used less often than the other devices, which creates placement problems. Position the mouse or other input devices centrally, and place your screen centrally or slightly to the side of your dominant eye. The large screen will require a lower position, and a keyboard tray will keep the keyboard central, but out of the way of the pointing device.

Many employees find themselves doing a combination of tasks—multitasking is the word you've heard—often sharing workstations with colleagues. Freelancers and office temps also move around from workplace to workplace. This type of work is the most difficult to set up for comfort. Learn your ideal workstation measurements, and carry a pocket tape measure so you can duplicate your personal measurements wherever you go. Avoid workplaces where there is no accommodation for some degree of ergonomic adjustment.

Serious Eye Problems

"Coal mines are no place for seventy-year-olds, but computer terminals are," said Senator Patrick Moynihan in 1999 on the lifting of earning limitations for Social Security recipients. The end of wage limitations means that older workers will be reentering the workforce as computer operators. As the workforce ages, these serious eye problems will become more common. The yearly eye examination to prevent or delay glaucoma, cataracts, and age-related macular degeneration is now more necessary than ever.

Glaucoma

The most common cause of blindness, glaucoma is an insidious illness that if detected in its early stages can be managed with medication to prevent progression.

Cataracts

A common cause of visual impairment, cataracts result from a clouding of the lens of the eye. As we age, cataracts become more common, and they advance more quickly if you have diabetes or have a long history of being exposed to ultraviolet light. Recent advances in treatment such as lens implants have helped to restore vision.

Age-Related Macular Degeneration

This serious illness has damaged the eyesight of 13 million Americans. Age-related macular degeneration affects people as early as their late fifties or sixties. Each year, 400,000 more Americans develop this serious problem. There is no known cure or lasting treatment. However, many devices are available to assist people with this condition, allowing them to continue to work on a limited basis.

Reading devices that magnify documents and project them onto a screen have been extremely helpful for the sight-impaired. Now there are LCD (liquid crystal display) technology projectors that hook up to computers that enlarge and project the monitor image onto a wall or screen. Large LCD or plasma screens now becoming more popular for TV use can also serve this purpose. These devices can be costly, but in some cases may give a legally blind person limited function at the computer.

Partially sighted people might make some use of voice-activated software, but such software still requires some keyboard use. Voice training is important to teach you how to enunciate properly, avoid slurring words, and speak more regularly as you dictate. Some software programs actually do this for you, but I usually recommend at least one session with a speech therapist, who can teach you to use your voice properly to prevent chronic hoarse voice. Placing the microphone properly is very important, as is recognizing the speed limitations of voice-activated software. Many systems are on the market, but a properly functioning system will need lots of RAM. There are several Internet Web sites that can guide you about what to buy, such as a voice users' group at http://www.voicerecognition.net.

5

Managing Pain

Nature has placed mankind under the governance of two sovereign masters, pain and pleasure.

–Jeremy Bentham, *Principles of Morals and Legislation*, 1789

Pain is the most common complaint in RSI, both in the early and late stages of the disorder, and it's the main reason why people come to see me. Pain tells us that injury is present, and it's a warning signal that shouldn't be ignored. Pain is something only *you* feel, and that's why it is difficult to convey its nature and intensity to others. This is especially true with RSI, because the afflicted person generally looks healthy–there are no open wounds. If your physician is insensitive or skeptical about your pain, you risk a worsening of your condition. Seek someone who cares, who will listen and help guide you to recovery. See the section on choosing a physician in chapter 2.

As RSI progresses, it becomes more obvious that the pain associated with it has variable qualities. It may start as a periodic aching associated with work and may become more severe, constant, and burning as time goes on. To make matters worse, other symptoms may arise, such as weakness, numbness, depression, anxiety, and panic. As RSI progresses, pain becomes more difficult to manage, a good reason to begin early treatment.

The most common type of pain is acute pain, which is usually temporary. It is our first line of defense against further injury. If you continue to work with acute pain, tendons, muscles, or joints may become inflamed. If you rest and obtain appropriate treatment, your acute pain usually goes away. Pain is an important message from your body, and one you must listen to. If you allow pain to progress unattended, you are in for trouble as it moves toward a chronic condition.

Most RSI victims suffer from one or more forms of chronic pain, which tend to persist long after the onset of an injury, and health care providers often mismanage chronic pain. Chronic pain can be dull one day and sharp another as it moves throughout the body. The good news is that it can eventually subside with appropriate treatment. If allowed to persist or worsen, a vicious cycle ensues, leading to a more complicated form of pain, complex chronic pain.

Complex chronic pain differs from acute or chronic pain because it stimulates a part of the nervous system called the limbic system. The limbic system is a group of brain structures common to all mammals and associated with involuntary nerve function, behavior, and smell. As RSI progresses, it can induce complex chronic pain by its effect on the sympathetic nervous system, over which we have little control. This dysfunction of the sympathetic nervous system perpetuates pain by beginning a vicious cycle of blood vessel instability accompanied by the release of pain-stimulating substances into the bloodstream that continue uncontrolled. Often it provokes the genesis of new pain fibers. One common sign of complex chronic pain is a cooling of the hands and forearms, often combined with sweating as the pain level increases. This is known as reflex sympathetic dysfunction. I have found this present in 20 percent of my RSI patients. When complex chronic pain occurs, treatment is usually more difficult and prolonged because circulatory changes diminish the blood supply to the soft tissues and delay healing.

Research suggests that this may be an early form of RSD/CRPS and may be more common than previously thought.

If aggressive and focused treatment is not begun quickly, the condition can progress to the most serious form of complex chronic pain, which is reflex sympathetic dystrophy (RSD) or complex regional pain syndrome (CRPS).

One of my patients is a good example of what can happen if RSD/CRPS is not recognized in time. M. L. is a university professor of literature who traveled from another city to see me. The use of a computer was an integral part of her work. A few months earlier, she had begun to notice the onset of pain and numbness in her right arm. For a month or so before this, she had spent long hours at her computer keyboard finishing a book. At first she felt pain only when working; later the pain persisted even after work. Finally it became a permanent part of her life, with worsening symptoms including a burning feeling. She saw her physician who, perplexed, recommended a second opinion. The second doctor suggested she stop using her arm, which had become by this time almost completely useless anyway. Her pain was so acute that she went around with her arm folded against her body so no one would accidentally touch it. She also noted that her hand and arm had become cold, and she could no longer continue her work. Her physician then suggested she wear a splint, which gave her some temporary relief. But in the long run, the splint compounded her problems. The immobilization told her brain that now her right extremity was completely shut down. Blood was shunted from the skin to the deeper tissues. Calcium was being washed out of the arm and hand bones, while skin and nail changes were beginning to become apparent. When I first saw her, she was in obvious pain, with her right arm flexed at the elbow. Her skin was dry and cool, except that her palms were sweaty. She complained of severe pain, which worsened when her skin was lightly touched. On further examination, I found that she had evidence of neurogenic thoracic outlet syndrome (see chapter 2) and a frozen right shoulder. I instructed her to discard her splint and begin moving her arm as much as she could tolerate it. I referred her to a physical therapist with a prescription to gradually mobilize her right arm and shoulder and begin postural retraining. Fortunately, her RSD/CRPS was still amenable to this approach. I also prescribed Neurontin (gabapentin; see later in this chapter) for her pain so that the therapist could begin manual work on her soft tissues. I kept in close contact with her and her physical therapist, monitoring her progress. It wasn't easy for M. L. to regain function, and the process took many months. But I was gratified to see marked improvement on her return visit. She was lucky after a year to have complete recovery, though I warned her to continue her mobility and strengthening exercises to avoid a relapse. Many other patients are not so fortunate.

Another young woman I saw came at a much later stage. Despite multiple interventions including nerve blocks, massage, and biofeedback, her RSD/CRPS spread to all her extremities, resulting in almost complete disability. To add to her woes, she entered a protracted battle with insurance carriers who seemed to have little understanding of the seriousness of her problem. Her prognosis for a return to health was poor.

In 1993, the term complex regional pain syndrome types 1 and 2 was proposed as a substitute for the term RSD by the International Association for the Study of Pain. Type 1 CRPS is essentially what we see in people with RSI who develop what was called RSD. The onset of type 1 CRPS is more closely related to soft-tissue injury than is type 2, which involves more severe nerve injury and was formerly called causalgia.

In both types there are four basic signs: Burning pain made worse by movement; swelling that is persistent and progressive and sometimes localized; stiffness that is progressive and results in diminished movement of the joints; and discoloration due to circulatory changes.

History and a physical examination usually can establish the diagnosis, especially when there are skin and temperature changes. The only early diagnostic tests that will produce findings are thermography or computer-assisted tomography, both of which are difficult to obtain. The other possible test is a stellate ganglion block, which consists of injecting a local anesthetic into the grouping of sympathetic nerves in the neck to see if this provides relief from pain. Yet it is at the early stage of this illness that aggressive treatment must begin. When the disease has reached a severe stage, tests such as MRI, EMG, and CT scans will show involvement of bone and soft tissues. But at this stage, treatment is far more difficult and less effective.

Treatment of RSD/CRPS

Early diagnosis can produce a good outcome. Begin physical therapy to maintain flexibility, range of motion, and strength. People with CRPS tend to limit movement because of stiffness and pain. They should be encouraged to perform range-of-motion exercises, but too vigorous an exercise program can cause a flare-up of symptoms. Use medications to control symptoms and to block sympathetic nerve overactivity. These include tricyclic antidepressants and gabapentin (Neurontin), which has proven to be especially effective. Sometimes other medications such as beta blockers, clonidine, and carbamazapine have been used. In more severe cases, nerve blocks may give temporary or permanent relief.

Make the necessary lifestyle changes, and provide ergonomic and biomechanical intervention. RSD/CRPS comprises about 10 percent to 20 percent of chronic pain patients. This means that there are approximately 4 million RSD/CRPS patients in the United States.

RSD/CRPS is a serious injury that must be recognized early and treated aggressively. RSD/CRPS can cause severe migraines, burning pain, swelling, nail changes, and movement disorders such as tremors and dystonia. It has been known to migrate to other body parts—for example, it can begin in one arm and then appear in the other arm or either or both legs. Any kind of soft-tissue injury, such as an operation causing nerve damage, or an injury as banal as getting your hand caught in a door, can lead to the onset of RSD/CRPS of the type 1 or type 2 variety (also see chapter 2).

In the RSI patient, the majority of whom have postural problems (rounded shoulders and head thrust forward), nerve injury from muscle imbalance combined with overuse of muscles are often enough to transform chronic pain into complex chronic pain because of sympathetic nervous system involvement. This may ultimately result in RSD/CRPS if treatment is not begun early enough to prevent it.

Self-Treatment

Learn from your pain, pay attention to your pain, and you should eventually conquer it. With RSI, rest may be the most important initial step toward healing. Here, rest is a relative term. Total rest, such as going to bed and lying there, quickly causes muscles to atrophy and contract. This is not the right type of rest. You need relative rest, avoiding anything that would stress your injured nerves and muscles. This means not only avoiding or diminishing computer use but also limiting other activities, such as playing musical instruments, knitting, gardening, cooking, or any upper-body activity that causes distress. While you may have to continue working to earn your living, you should take rest breaks, pace yourself, and stretch during the workday. This means you may have to negotiate with your supervisor (or yourself) about your work pace. After making certain ergonomic and biomechanical changes and getting medically evaluated, you are ready to begin working with your physical or occupational therapist to conquer RSI.

Icing is an immediate and effective way to diminish the level of pain in RSI. It is most effective if the ice is put in direct contact with the skin for short intervals of forty to sixty seconds. It should be applied by moving it over painful tissues until the skin gets slightly numb and reddish. Do this for no more than a minute at a time and no more than ten times a day. Don't stretch the iced muscle because muscles tend to gel when cold. Wait at least fifteen minutes before you begin gentle stretching. Do not use ice until you have consulted with your physician. Do not use ice if you have reflex sympathetic dysfunction or RSD/CRPS, or if you have circulatory problems, diabetes, Raynaud's syndrome, or any other condition where cold might be harmful.

An easy way to apply ice is to fill a paper cup with water and let it freeze. When it is solid, tear off the lip, place your arm on a towel and apply it directly to the skin, rubbing back and forth gently. Place the cup back in the freezer for reuse.

Although it is usually not as effective as ice in relieving pain, heat can relax soft tissues, even though it doesn't penetrate very deeply. You can apply heat in a variety of ways, including a heating pad, moist hot packs, and a warm shower. Your therapist can use ultrasound. Avoid high levels of heat and prolonged application, since these can produce burns and skin mottling or discoloration.

Some treating physicians recommend application of topical creams and liquids to diminish muscle pain. These are aspirin-based creams, NSAID creams, and creams containing capsaicin. Capsaicin is a pepper derivative, and its use should be limited to two days at a time to avoid dermatitis, blistering, and ulceration.

Transcutaneous Electrical Nerve Stimulator (TENS)

TENS is a noninvasive electrical device that stimulates the nerve fibers that travel to the neocortex of the brain. It is used for controlling pain at trigger points and is helpful particularly in the treatment of RSD/CRPS by applying stimulation at multiple locations.

Acupuncture and Acupressure

Acupuncture is a treatment that involves sticking small needles into key parts of the body that relate to the symptoms' sites. Acupressure involves applying hand pressure to these sites. Acupuncture is useful for the treatment of pain driven by an overactive sympathetic nervous system (complex chronic pain) and works best for that condition by stimulating specific nerve fibers. One of its effects is to activate endorphins, which are the body's natural pain suppressors.

Acupuncture is not a very useful treatment for simple chronic pain because it provides relief that lasts for only a few hours. Acupuncture is less effective if used as the sole therapy modality and should be used in conjunction with occupational and physical therapy. Acupuncture should be performed only by qualified, experienced practitioners.

Local Injections of Corticosteroids and Anesthetics

Some physicians, to relieve acute tendinitis or other inflammations such as painful trigger points, use local injections of solutions containing steroids or a local anesthetic. These injections can break the pain cycle and diminish inflammation. Steroid injections should be limited to no more than two or three applications at one site, since they can potentially cause tendon rupture, which could need surgical repair. Steroid injections can dissolve fatty tissue, leaving unsightly pitted areas in the skin.

In the hands of experienced and competent physicians, these injections can be helpful. Systemic side effects from corticosteroids can occur, which might include rising blood sugar, muscle weakness, osteoporosis, or increased susceptibility to infection.

Iontophoresis and Phonophoresis

Corticosteroids also can be applied in less traumatic ways. Local areas of inflammation can be reduced by applying a 10 percent hydrocortisone cream to the skin and driving it into the tissues with an electric current (iontophoresis) or with sound waves (phonophoresis). This is usually prescribed by a physician but performed by a physical or occupational therapist.

Splints

The use of splints to control pain is usually a step in the wrong direction. Most of the injury and pain associated with RSI needs to heal actively. By this I mean that some gentle movement is necessary to encourage soft tissues to grow with the lines of force (proper direction) of the tissue. Immobilizing these tissues might relieve some of your pain, but splinting will simply encourage muscle weakness and random, chaotic tissue healing that will be less functional than the tissue was before the injury. Furthermore, with splinting, joints become stiff and muscles atrophy. More seriously, the immobilization of splinting can lead to, worsen, or predispose you to RSD/CRPS. If you have a broken bone, a splint or a cast is a logical treatment, but when it's removed, the immobilized soft tissues always need to be rehabilitated. Unfortunately, too many physicians and therapists treat soft-tissue injury as if they were treating a broken bone, which can prolong the problem.

Many people splint themselves in a misguided attempt to prevent RSI or to keep it from developing or spreading. Wrist splints may cause pain to migrate to muscles that have not been immobilized by the splint. This increases muscle imbalance by causing atrophy in one group of muscles and overuse in another. If you are concerned about keeping your wrists straight, don't do it with a splint. Instead, get a split keyboard, change your technique, and check the ergonomics of your workstation. See chapters 7 and 8 for more details.

Occasionally, splinting may be necessary to overcome a severe, acute inflammation such as the thumb tendinitis of DeQuervain's disease or to get relief from night pain if you are suffering from carpal tunnel syndrome. If your doctor gives you splints, ask what the rationale for the treatment is. Always use splints for the minimum amount of time, and never splint yourself. Recently a physical therapist I know, competent and aware of the dangers of splinting, applied a short-term splint for someone with acute DeQuervain's disease. In a week, the patient developed early signs of RSD/CRPS. Thanks to the awareness and quick action of the therapist, treatment was started immediately, but it took almost a year for the symptoms to subside completely.

Mental Splinting

Mental splinting means that you make a knowledgeable attempt to minimize injury by using proper technique. To do this you should be at a point in your therapy where you have enough strength to do this and you are free of pain. Your therapist can help you by guiding you in proper ergonomics and biomechanics.

Drug Treatment of Acute Pain

Acute pain in RSI usually results from an acute inflammatory reaction of soft tissues to trauma, such as a tendon under tension, (golfer's or tennis elbow), a tendon rubbing against its sheath (DeQuervain's disease), or acute low-back syndrome. Apart from measures such as ergonomic intervention, icing, rest, stretching, and gentle soft tissue work by a therapist, a number of anti-inflammatory medications are often prescribed. These should be used cautiously, and under a physician's supervision. Medications to treat acute pain and inflammation are a big business for the pharmaceutical industry, and there are a large number of products with similar characteristics and risks. They tend to give limited relief in chronic pain, work better for acute pain, and often are costly.

Nonsteroidal Anti-inflammatory Medications (NSAIDs)

There are many anti-inflammatory and pain relief medications available either over the counter or by prescription that give a certain amount of relief of acute pain. Since most RSI patients suffer from chronic pain, NSAIDs are likely to give only partial relief.

NSAIDs are the most frequently used medication worldwide. This has led to the realization that the complications of NSAIDs use, particularly when used on a continuing basis, can be serious. One of the more dangerous effects is on the gastrointestinal tract, where bleeding and ulceration can occur. The liver, kidneys, and the cardiovascular system can also be adversely affected, especially in the elderly. Moreover, not all NSAIDs have the same toxicity profile. These potential complications have sparked research in a quest for a safer NSAID derivative.

NSAIDs work by inhibiting the so-called cyclooxygenase systems (COX). Two main COX systems were found to be inhibited by NSAIDs. This led to a separation of NSAIDs into two categories—conventional and gastroprotective— based on their effect on the COX systems.

Conventional NSAIDs

diclofenac (Voltaren, Cataflam)
mefenamic acid (Ponstel)
diflunisal (Dolobid)
meloxicam (Mobic)
etodolac (Lodine)
naproxen (Naprosyn, Anaprox, Naprelan)
fenoprofen (Nalfon)
piroxicam (Feldene)
ibuprofen (Motrin, Vicoprofen)
salsalate (Disalcid)
indomethacin (Indocin)
sulindac (Clinoril)
ketoprofen (Orudis, Oruvail)
tolmetin sodium (Tolectin)
ketorolac tromethamine (Toradol, Acular)

The COX-1 system is found mostly in the gastrointestinal tract and is said to have a protective function, particularly in preventing peptic ulcers and hemorrhage. The COX-2 system is found at the site of an inflammatory reaction, where it produces prostaglandins. Therefore, finding a specific COX-2 inhibitor would be desirable, since its main effect would be to diminish inflammation and pain without endangering the gastrointestinal system and kidneys. Two approaches have been developed to solve the problem. The rationale involves trying to selectively inhibit COX-2 activity and benefiting from its analgesic and anti-inflammatory activity, while allowing the COX-1 system to carry on its protective function in the gastric mucosa and kidneys.

Two COX-2 specific inhibitors have been in use since 1998. They are celecoxib (Celebrex) and rofecoxib (VIOXX). A third medication, nabumetone (Relafen) may also have high COX-2 capability. Another approach to these potential complications is to combine a conventional NSAID, diclofenac (Voltaren, Cataflam) with misoprostol (Arthrotec), a drug that increases production of bicarbonate and mucus and decreases acid production, thus offering protection from bleeding and other complications.

Gastroprotective NSAIDs

celecoxib (Celebrex)
rofecoxib (VIOXX)
nambutone (Relaflex)
diclofenac and misoprostol (Arthrotec)

Finally, there is a potential conflict between at least one NSAID—ibuprofen (Advil)—and aspirin. Advil diminishes the cardiac-protective effect of aspirin. Also, if you are taking an ACE inhibitor for high blood pressure, you should avoid NSAIDs.

A severe life-threatening condition known as an anaphylactoid reaction can occur with NSAID and aspirin use. This can present as an acute allergic reaction preceded by a sense of uneasiness, agitation, and flushing, then tingling, itching, difficulty breathing, convulsions, and shock. Immediate medical care in such cases is essential.

It should be noted that the whole area of NSAIDs and their

complex relationships with the COX systems is undergoing further intensive evaluation by researchers. NSAIDs and NSAID derivatives are useful, but they should be used with great care, based on the treating physician's decision. Even with gastroprotective NSAIDs there is still some risk of GI bleeding, which can increase with the simultaneous use of SSRI antidepressant medication.

Aspirin and Other Salicylates

Aspirin is a salicylate that has many actions, including the ability to reduce pain, fever, and inflammation. Like NSAIDs, it inhibits COX-1 and COX-2 systems. The risks are similar to those of NSAIDs, including the potential for allergic reactions. Aspirin is often compounded with codeine or codeine derivatives to make it a more effective pain medication because codeine desensitizes the nerves to all pain-stimulating substances, not only prostaglandins. Aspirin can also be applied locally in the form of a cream. Choline magnesium trisalicylate (Trisilate) is similar to aspirin in its action. Consult your physician before using any of these medications, and avoid them if you are pregnant.

Other Pain Medications

Acetaminophen has fewer side effects than aspirin, although it should not be taken with heavy alcohol use. It is often combined with codeine to block the pain-producing substances linked to RSI. It is a weak nonselective inhibitor of COX-1 and COX-2. It is not an NSAID, and it has a low incidence of gastrointestinal complications. It provides pain relief but has no anti-inflammatory effect. There are various brands of acetaminophen, but there is little if any difference among them.

Muscle Relaxants

There is a group of medications whose purpose is to relieve muscle spasm. They also provide analgesia, which in some cases may be better than aspirin or acetaminophen. Side effects may include headache, diarrhea, drowsiness, and dry mouth.

Muscle Relaxants

chlorzoxazone (Paraflex, Parafon Forte, Remular-S)
carisoprodol (Soma)
cyclobenzaprine HCL (Flexeril)
methocarbamol (Robaxin)
orphenadrine citrate (Norflex, Norgesic)

Orphenadrine citrate is prescribed to relieve mild to moderate musculoskeletal pain. It should be avoided if you have glaucoma, bladder or prostate problems, or an allergy to aspirin. Norflex is sometimes prescribed as a muscle relaxant. These medications, while useful, have many potential side effects and should only be taken after careful assessment of your ability to tolerate them safely.

The Antidepressants' Role in Pain Management

Recent investigations in sports medicine have shown that after an injury, athletes often suffer a period of depression. Depression and anxiety are common parts of RSI. Aside from treating depression, antidepressants raise the pain threshold and are often used in conjunction with NSAIDs and physical therapy to control pain. The two main classes of antidepressants used in pain management are the tricyclics and the selective serotonin reuptake inhibitors (SSRIs). The tricyclics are particularly useful in controlling complex chronic pain.

The tricyclic group includes medications such as amitryptyline and nortriptyline HCL (Aventyl) and desipramine (Norpramin). The tricyclics are used for chronic pain management in RSI, although they have many side effects and interact with a number of other substances, including monoamine oxidase inhibitors, yet another class of drugs used in the treatment of depression. These side effects include cardiac arrhythmias, postural hypotension (a drop in blood pressure when moving from a sitting to a standing position), sedation (drowsiness,) dry mouth, constipation, confusion, and urinary retention. Tricyclics relieve pain through serotonin and norepinephrine reuptake blockade as well as blockade of alpha receptors and sodium channels. (See the glossary.) Tricyclic antidepressants are the first line in the medicinal treatment of RSD/CRPS.

The selective serotonin reuptake inhibitors are a newer group of antidepressants, and include fluoxetine HCL (Prozac), sertraline HCL (Zoloft), paroxetine HCL (Paxil), and citalopram (Celexa). They are sometimes used with NSAIDs because they raise the pain threshold, but they are not as effective as tricyclics in the management of chronic pain. Unrelated chemically to tricyclics, these antidepressants block central nervous system uptake of serotonin. They are also used to treat anxiety, panic disorder, and obsessive-compulsive disorder. These medications to control pain and depression should only be taken under the direction of a psychiatrist who specializes in psychopharmacology.

Recently there has been some concern about the finding that SSRIs can increase the risk of gastrointestinal bleeding. The relative risk has been described as being about three times higher than in persons not on SSRIs. Although the absolute risk is small, it is increased if patients are on NSAIDs or aspirin. Apparently SSRIs inhibit the uptake of platelet serotonin, weakening the blood's ability to clot.

Gabapentin (Neurontin)

Recently this second-generation antiepilepsy drug has been found promising as a medication to control neuropathic pain associated with RSI and several other conditions, including RSD/CRPS. The way gabapentin works is not fully understood, but it is distinct from the way that the tricyclics and SSRIs work and is proving to be a very useful medication because it is well tolerated with few side effects. It is, however, expensive.

For many persons undergoing the initial stages of treatment

who cannot tolerate soft-tissue work, Neurontin is useful to diminish pain and allow the therapist to perform necessary deep-tissue work. The dosage of Neurontin will vary according to what your physician feels is optimal. High doses may be necessary in some people to get an optimal therapeutic effect. Side effects include sleepiness and dizziness. As with any other of these medications, Neurontin should be used only if necessary and for as short a time as possible.

Carbamazepine (Tegretol, Carbetrol)

Carbamazepine is an anticonvulsant and specific analgesic used to treat trigeminal neuralgia (a painful inflammation of a nerve in the face). It is sometimes used in the treatment of RSD/CRPS in combination with physical therapy. However, there are other medications, such as gabapentin, that produce the same results with fewer side effects. Its mechanism of action is unclear. Agranulocytosis, a serious blood disorder, has been reported with Tegretol, which should be used with care.

Clonidine (Catapres) and Tizanidine (Zanaflex)

These are both adrenergic antagonists. Clonidine is generally used for the treatment of high blood pressure. Because it acts on the central nervous system to reduce sympathetic nerve activity, it has been used in the treatment of RSD/CRPS.

Tizanidine is useful in the treatment of headache and neuropathic pain. These drugs should be carefully titrated. Side effects include sedation, hypotension, and dry mouth.

Propanolol (Inderal)

Propanolol is a beta adrenergic receptor blocking agent used in the treatment of hypertension and cardiovascular disease. It diminishes sympathetic nerve effect and has been used in the treatment of RSD/CRPS. Tricyclics, serotonin reuptake inhibitors, and gabapentin (Neurontin) are now more likely to be the drugs of choice. Propanolol is sometimes prescribed for performers and speakers to control performance anxiety or stage fright.

Opioid-Based Medications

The most useful of these are codeine, oxycodone, and propoxyphene napsylate (Darvocet, Darvon-N, and Propacet, respectively). Usually these medications are combined with NSAIDs or aspirin to produce a greater beneficial effect than each would do alone. The opioids can counteract most of the pain-stimulating substances released from injured tissues. Opioids have limited long-term use because of significant side effects such as dizziness, nausea, constipation, the need for increasing doses over time, and the possibility of habituation. Habituation is less likely if severe pain is present and sustained. Opioids relieve pain through activation of a number of specific receptors found in both the central and peripheral nervous systems.

Oxycontin

Special attention should be focused on a form of oxycodone called Oxycontin. Recently, the potential for abuse and fatal overdose has been reported. Since this is a slow-release tablet, it should be swallowed whole, and not broken or crushed, which causes a sudden release that can be fatal. This drug should be used only in people who are opioid-tolerant. There is little if any indication to use this medication in RSI.

Chondroitin Sulfate and Glucosamine

Recently, a combination of chondroitin sulfate and glucosamine has received attention as a medication for treating arthritis, rebuilding cartilage, and diminishing pain indirectly. Although many people find it helpful, reliable scientific proof of its efficacy is not yet available. Studies are being conducted to determine its usefulness.

Physical Therapy, Occupational Therapy, and Home Exercises

Stretching, strengthening, postural exercises, and soft-tissue work under the guidance of your therapist are the front-line defenses against pain and ultimately the bases for healing and resolution of RSI. The supply system for these defenses is your conscientious attention to your home program, so that, without backsliding, progress is made each time you see a therapist. The team approach to treatment can't be overemphasized. In some cases, additional therapeutic modalities can augment your treatment team's work but should not substitute for it.

6

Your Lower Back

Our torments may also in length of time become our elements.

–John Milton (1608–1674), *Paradise Lost*

Good posture is essential in preventing repetitive strain injury, and your lower back is the foundation on which the many other elements of posture are built. If you sit at your computer for long periods of time, you may think you are not doing much physical work. Yet the muscles of your lower back are hard at work maintaining you in this seated position. The kind of physical work your muscles are doing is defined as static loading, where the muscles act as braces for your frame. Static loading also forces these muscles to work with less nourishment in the form of blood supply, and therefore they are more vulnerable to fatigue. This is more likely to occur if you are poorly conditioned, or if you assume awkward postures as a result of poor workstation equipment or arrangement.

It is estimated that 50 to 80 percent of people in developed countries suffer from lower back pain. Next to upper body RSI, low back syndrome is the most frequent work-related problem reported to employers as a cause of disability.

Your occupation may not be the only reason you incur low back pain. As in upper body repetitive strain, there are many possible causes, and this creates confusion. Some of the risk factors relate to what you do and how you do it at home. Other elements of your lifestyle, such as the sports you engage in, your physical condition, and your diet can also become risk factors. Things not necessarily under your control, such as your hereditary makeup, your age, your sex, or an underlying illness play a role as well. Static or awkward posture, anxiety, mental stress, depression, and job dissatisfaction are all strong risk factors.

Because of its sheer number of victims, lower back pain has become a serious socioeconomic problem, costing industry and the health care system billions of dollars annually. In the United States, approximately $14 billion a year are spent dealing with the results of lower back pain. To put it in personal terms, every adult has an episode of low back pain at least three times in his or her life.

Our bipedal posture places great vertical and lateral pressure on the spine. This can result in two common injuries. The first, spondylolysis, accounts for 6 percent of low back pain. This condition results from a defect in function of the superior and inferior articular processes (see chapter 1), usually of the fourth and fifth lumbar vertebrae. As much as 50 percent of athletes with low back pain may be suffering from spondylolysis.

Another mechanical condition that might occur is called spondylolisthesis. Here, there is slippage of the body of the vertebra above another vertebra. This typically occurs as a result of degenerative changes in the spine—rheumatoid arthritis or osteoarthritis, for example.

Defining Low Back Pain

Low back pain exists under a number of different names: lumbago, painful lumbar syndrome, lumbosacral strain, or sciatica if the sciatic nerve root is involved. If acute pain persists for twelve weeks or more, it can be considered chronic.

Apart from bony involvement by deterioration or slippage of spinal elements, pain in the lower back is usually the pain of muscle spasm, where nerve fibers are irritated by a tightened muscle. There is associated stiffness and increased pain on certain movements. This pain usually has no recognizable pathology—you rarely find an infection, a fracture, or a tumor. Fortunately, 90 percent of people recover from acute low back pain in about six weeks. Between 2 and 7 percent of those with acute low back pain evolve into chronic pain. Recurrent pain attacks account for the majority of absenteeism from work.

In upper body RSI, we know that the pain is subjective—you are the only one who can experience it and discern its characteristics and intensity. This can create problems for patients, since the examining physician may not understand or believe what the victim is experiencing. This is when many people are told that "it's all in your mind." The same is true for low back pain. The subjective nature of the pain may also make it difficult to treat. Objective evidence can often be elicited by applying pressure to the painful area and noting the sudden reaction of the patient—he or she might exclaim, jump, or whine.

Poor work habits are generally the main cause of low back pain. Specifically, about 70 percent of the pain is associated with sudden or heavy lifting, usually done improperly with the legs extended instead of bent. Pushing or pulling can account for another 10 to 15 percent of injury. Don't consider yourself immune just because your work doesn't usually include these activities. If you are in poor general condition, inadvertent lifting or pushing (even just reaching for the filing cabinet) can set off an acute episode. Simply sitting at your workstation can place substantial demands on your lower back. Other activities you may not even realize put you at risk may bring on an episode: jogging, aerobics, tennis, golf. Even eating to excess can cause you to gain weight that places an extra burden not only on the spine, but on the hips and knees as well. If you are a musician playing the cello or other instrument while sitting, you are at risk. If your instrument is played standing, you may also be at risk. I've treated numerous percussion and bass players whose low back static tension led to their problems. Sometimes the cause of these events can be extremely difficult to detect. As an examining physician, a thorough history and physical examination or even a biomechanical and ergonomic analysis may be the kind of detective work needed.

X-rays and MRIs are usually ordered by the examining physician, who must avoid the trap of considering any single finding as the cause of the problem. Many people with abnormal X-rays may have no symptoms at all. In fact, about 85 percent of people will have no discernible finding. About 4 percent of the time, compression fractures related to falls and osteoporosis are found, while about 1 percent are found to have spinal tumors.

Treatment of Acute Low Back Pain

Acute low back pain may be treated differently from the chronic variety. Acute low back pain is essentially a self-limiting disease. In the past, bed rest was a treatment mainstay, easily accepted by patients for the obvious reason that it affords immediate relief. It is now recognized, however, that continued activity is not harmful, and is in fact the best way to promote healing. Bed rest can be harmful in that it can stiffen or weaken muscles that need to be mobilized and used. During the acute period, NSAIDs (see chapter 5) can be useful to control pain and facilitate activity. Muscle relaxants can also be helpful, but they have side effects including sleepiness and habituation potential for some. Behavioral therapy that consists of working with a professional to resolve issues such as anxiety and fear can also help. Ergonomic and biomechanical interventions are appropriate as well during this stage.

On the other hand, there are approaches that may have minimal or doubtful effectiveness. Often these approaches may not be harmful in themselves, but they may not be cost-effective. These include the use of certain strong analgesics such as opioids, antidepressants, colchicine (a drug used for its anti-inflammatory effects), steroid injections, facet joint injections, trigger point injections, biofeedback, massage, traction, spinal manipulation, acupuncture, and lumbar supports. The decision to use one or more of these approaches should be made in consultation with your physician or physical therapist, since some might be helpful in specific cases.

Treatment of Chronic Low Back Pain

In chronic cases, exercise therapy becomes a cornerstone of treatment, which should include strengthening the often forgotten abdominals. Changing the working milieu with ergonomic and biomechanical interventions is useful. Likely to be beneficial are behavioral therapy, the use of NSAIDs and analgesics, trigger point injections, and attending a back school. Back schools—programs usually administered by the physiatry department of a hospital or a back pain center—teach you both preventive and treatment aspects of low back pain. The knowledge gained can be extremely helpful in improving conditions. There is less unanimity about certain other measures, but they may be useful in specific cases. These include using antidepressants and muscle relaxants, epidural steroid injections, and lumbar supports. Transcutaneous electrical nerve stimulation (TENS) to block pain messages, spinal manipulation, and acupuncture are also sometimes used. Two approaches that are either ineffective or harmful are facet joint injections and traction.

Surgery for Back Pain

Surgery for back pain is a minefield of controversy. Of course, if diagnostic tests reveal the presence of a specific lesion, such as a tumor, or if there is a progressive neurological deficit, surgery may be the solution. But in the absence of such findings, surgery can be a problem. Immobilizing spinal segments may possibly relieve some of the pain, but it can also upset the delicate dynamic of the spinal column. Still, some people are willing to accept less function for relief from pain. If surgery is contemplated, seek at least a second opinion and look for a physician who has experience with low back surgery. Often the decision about what kind of physician should do this surgery comes up, since both orthopedic surgeons and neurosurgeons may be adept at it.

Low back pain is a common, and often neglected, component of the diagnosis and treatment of RSI. Simply understanding the reasons for its onset and the possible treatments can be helpful in obtaining relief.

7

Physical and Occupational Therapy for RSI

I bend and I break not.

–Jean de la Fontaine (1621–1695)

Physical and occupational therapy are the keystones of care in repetitive strain injury. Once you have been diagnosed with RSI, the treatment portion of your therapy should begin. To regain what you have lost in normal body function, you must concentrate on your body. This means total attention to your therapist's instructions and your home program. Anything less prolongs your pain and your other symptoms. In most cases, treatment must begin gradually to avoid relapse. This is where your therapist becomes indispensable.

A common mistake at the beginning of therapy is to overdo it. Another is the false belief that without pain there is no gain. In RSI, pain should never be used as a guide to exercise progression. You must rely on your own awareness. Relying on the therapist to carry the workload of your recovery means that you will not recover. Your home program is what maintains your therapist's mobilization effort while taking you to your next level of progress. And once you are better, you will maintain that condition only if you change your exercise habits permanently. Getting back to work requires constant vigilance in your exercise program. You can never return to indolence if you want to stay healthy.

The Right Therapy with the Right Therapist

You won't recover from RSI unless you work hard at it. There is no quick fix or easy way out. This means participating in a program of exercises and other treatments under the guidance of your physician and your physical or occupational therapist. This chapter describes both basic and advanced exercises and stretches, most of which you can do at home, at work, and in the gym on a regular basis with the periodic supervision of your therapist. This sounds easy enough, but it is a major challenge to find not only the right physician (see chapter 2) but the right therapist as well.

Finding Treatment

The person in charge of your therapy should be a certified physical or occupational therapist with a bona fide interest in RSI. This is not a job for the trainer at your gym. Find out whether the facility you're considering is a busy one—your therapist will need to spend a lot of personal time with you. Visit the facility and note how much time the therapist spends with each client.

Beware of the therapist who insists on the immediate use of weight training. Premature use of weights will only add to your symptoms, and this is one of the principal reasons why patients abandon treatment. You should not be using weights for forearm and wrist exercises when you start treatment, but only after healing has begun and your forearm and wrist pains have diminished. If your therapist doesn't understand this principle, find someone who does. Poor management by the therapist can make you cynical about therapy and delay your recovery, and rotating therapists is not the best approach. You need to develop a relationship with one supervising therapist; any substitute should be part of your primary therapist's team.

Personal Trainers

Personal trainers who often work in gyms are not qualified to treat RSI. In a recent study done at Lehman College in New York City, a survey of 247 trainers revealed that 20 percent of them had no certification whatsoever. Trainers may be fine for the healthy, and many trainers are quite knowledgeable. But RSI is a serious medical condition. Trainers should not be considered a substitute for your physical or occupational therapist. Once your condition improves, a competent trainer could work with your therapist to continue your ongoing maintenance program.

Fight for Therapy Coverage

Unfortunately, managed care, workers' compensation, and restricted insurance reimbursement have curtailed benefits for physical and occupational therapy. This therapy is important, and you should go to great lengths to secure your coverage benefits. Do not accept rejection of therapy claims without battling for what is a necessary and vital part of your treatment. Often, your insurance provider just does not understand RSI. Enlist your physician, therapist, benefits manager, and anyone else who can help you document your needs. Don't give up!

Why You Need Your Exercise Program

Proper exercise is as critical to you as it is to a professional athlete. If you are recovering from RSI injury without active participation in home or gym exercises, you are not likely to get completely better. The same holds true if you want to prevent RSI. A physician and physical or occupational therapist working together is the best approach to your exercise program. Too much exercise or inappropriate exercise may increase pain or aggravate symptoms. Too little exercise could impede the progress of treatment.

A regular exercise program is important if you want to get rid of the pain, numbness, tingling, and disability of the disorder. Remember: you are an upper body athlete. Any athlete needs training to use his or her body. None of the following exercises should be done without a physical examination by a physician, who should provide a prescription for the therapist based on your examination findings. These exercises are a guide for your therapist and must be supervised by him or her. Self-programming your exercise regimen could lead to injury, which could undermine your will to continue this essential part of your therapy.

The RSI Exercise Program

Warm-ups

Warm-ups are a critical prelude to your exercise program. Warm-ups enhance circulation and mobilization of the soft tissues, maximizing the benefits of the rest of your exercise program.

Wall angels

No gym equipment is necessary here. Wall angels, which can be done against a wall or on the floor, mobilize the joints of the upper back, shoulders, and neck, increasing mobility and circulation. Any flat wall surface or floor area will do. The legs should be held slightly apart, the knees bent, and the back and arms flat against the wall or floor. The abdomen should be tucked in slightly. As you move your arms up and down, you will feel the shoulder blades moving and loosening, without the use of your upper trapezius muscles (between the neck and the shoulder). This exercise is harder to do than it looks, but gradually will

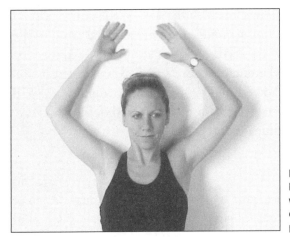

Done against the wall or lying on the floor, this warm-up exercise is also excellent for correcting posture.

become easier as your posture improves. Start with one or two sets of five wall angels two or three times daily, adding sets based on the advice of your therapist.

The UBE (Upper Body Ergometer)

This device is available in some gyms. If you are lucky enough to have access to one, it is an excellent upper body warm-up device. Properly used, the UBE will exercise the large trunk muscles instead of the smaller forearm muscles. The shoulder

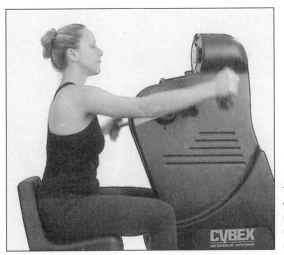

The UBE is a good warm-up apparatus that later can also promote upper back and shoulder mobility and strength.

joint should be lined up with the axis of the crank of the UBE. Resistance is set at a minimum level, and the handles are held loosely. Use of the UBE should be under the counsel of your therapist to determine time limits and to avoid the possibility of further injury. You should have assistance in fitting the UBE for your proportions prior to use, and you should memorize these settings for the future.

Bodyblade

This is a device you can purchase for home use, since it is generally not available in gyms. It comes in two sizes. Start with the smaller length. Basically, Bodyblade is a flexible bow with a handle in the middle that makes the blade oscillate when you shake it. Initially, you use Bodyblade by shaking it and changing direction frequently, which encourages natural muscle function. It is not as easy to master as it appears, and injured persons should start with thirty seconds of use, building up to three to six minutes with the supervision of the therapist.

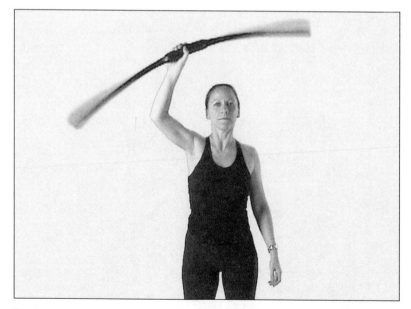

Bodyblade is also a good warm-up device that subsequently can be used to strengthen upper body muscles.

General Body Warm-up

Bicycle Warm-up

The stationary bicycle can substitute as a warm-up device, improving circulation in the entire body. Virtually all gyms have them; you may even have one at home. Holding the handlebars tightly while doing the warm-ups should be avoided because gripping the bars could cause a flare-up of your injury. Stationary bikes with wide seats are easier to pedal without holding the handlebars. Since you use only the lower body in this exercise, beginners have greater tolerance to this warm-up.

Running and Walking

Slow running and walking are excellent total body warm-up exercises. Your arms should be slightly flexed at chest level and moved while you walk or run, to mobilize your shoulders. Some people have difficulty with this exercise because they cannot tolerate the strain on their arms. Seek the guidance of your therapist regarding this warm-up; it may not be the best one for you.

Stretches

Stretching the soft tissues prepares them for mobilization and strengthening. Stretching can improve muscle balance and diminish the pressure on nerves, joints, and other structures. Stretching should be done regularly and become an integral part of your treatment or prevention program. A stretch should be held for a minimum of thirty seconds to be effective.

Before beginning your stretches the guidance of your physician or therapist is essential to determine which of your joints are hypermobile and which are tight. The hypermobile joints should not be overstretched, since this could cause a reactive muscle tightness or spasm. Wrist stretches are necessary for tightened forearm muscles in people with RSI. Conditions such as carpal tunnel syndrome can improve slowly if stretching and soft-tissue work by your therapist are combined. Stretching should be done twice a day or more. Stretching during your rest breaks can lead to a regular routine that becomes a good habit.

Trapezius and scalene stretches

It is very important to consult your physician about neck stretches. While most of the patients I have seen have neurogenic thoracic outlet syndrome accompanied by tightened neck muscles, a small percentage have protruding discs in the neck. This is a condition known as cervical radiculopathy, and stretching might aggravate it, so consult your physician before you decide to embark on neck stretches.

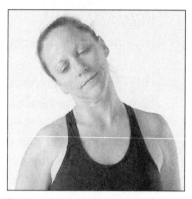

To stretch trapezius and scalene muscles, gently tuck your chin in toward your chest and depress the shoulder opposite to the one you are stretching. Placing the arm on the side being stretched behind your back helps to depress the shoulder on that side. Look straight ahead before beginning the stretch, and don't force the stretch by pushing hard on your head.

This important stretching exercise conditions the neck, back, and shoulder muscles, preparing them for strengthening and relieving pressure on nerves in the neck.

Wrist flexor stretches

These can be performed many times a day, especially during rest breaks. If you are double-jointed at the elbow, perform the flexor stretch with the elbow flexed to ninety degrees. Push with the other hand on the palm, not on the fingers.

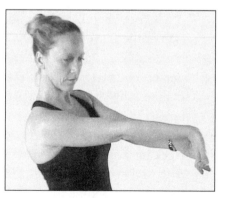

It is important to stretch the forearm flexor muscles as shown. If you are double-jointed at the elbow, perform this stretch with the elbow at a ninety-degree angle.

Wrist extensor stretches

Wrist extensor stretches are performed with the arm extended. Keep the shoulder down on the side you are stretching.

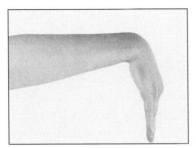

Stretching the forearm extensor muscle

Physioball/Resist-a-ball exercises

Most gyms have inflatable balls of various sizes that can be helpful for stretching certain difficult-to-get-at muscle groups. It is probably best to start with the largest size. The illustration below shows the ball being used to stretch the spine while side-lying. You may lie with your back arching over the ball to stretch your spine and abdominal muscles. For lower trapezius development and improvement of range of motion, lie face down on the ball and perform swimming strokes. There are other focused stretches to get at certain muscle groups that can be done with the ball; speak to your therapist about them. The ball should be used under the supervision of your therapist, who also can tell you what size ball you should use.

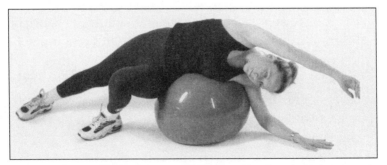

The air-filled heavy plastic ball is very useful for stretching the spinal column muscles.

Other stretches

There are many beneficial stretches, particularly those that increase spinal mobility. These should not be performed without consulting your physician or therapist.

Strengthening Exercises

After your initial evaluation, strengthening exercises usually begin with two sets of ten exercises, twice a day. These exercises should be tailored to your needs. At the beginning of strengthening exercises, do not use any weights. If soreness is experienced after exercises but does not continue into the next day, you may safely continue, but if soreness lasts into the following day, your exercises were too intense. In that case you should back off to one set of exercises twice daily.

Weights should be added to your program with caution, as they can cause injury if you are not prepared to tolerate them, and they should not be used until you can tolerate two sets of exercises twice a day. Weights should never be increased by more than half a pound per week.

If you have pain at rest in your hands or forearms, start with a cuff weight, not a dumbbell weight. There are cuff weights with pockets that take metal rods so you can gradually increase the weight. As pain decreases, switch to dumbbells, holding them lightly rather than gripping them.

Pain is a signal not to be ignored.

Muscle soreness or a sense of weakness (not pain) indicates that you are approaching your limit. With the guidance of your therapist, a few more repetitions beyond this sensation of weakness may help you to move to a higher level of effort.

Make sure your therapist is documenting your progress. This should include an RSI log that documents both your progress and pain severity (using a 1–10 scale) This is easy to do with your therapist's help.

The principles outlined above can also be applied to activities of daily living at home, which are discussed in chapter 10.

For example, if pain from any home activity carries over to the next day, you are doing too much. Back off.

The Basic 5

These exercises can help you begin the process of healing. For side-lying exercises you can use a pillow under your arm or trunk to elevate your body and decrease pressure on your shoulder.

Punching the ceiling (superior serratus anterior muscle)

Lying flat on your back, raise both arms toward the ceiling. Hold for three seconds. Lower each arm slowly and avoid elevating your shoulders. Attempt to do them twice a day, ten repetitions, advancing to multiple sets of ten. If pain continues to the next day, discontinue and discuss with your therapist.

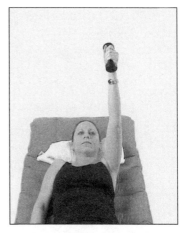

The "punching the ceiling" exercise should be started without weights.

Side-lying whole arm raises (perform on both sides)

Lie on your side, with the top arm elbow extended. Raise and lower the arm so the palm touches the floor. If this maneuver causes increased irritation in the elbow, try lowering the arm only halfway. Attempt these twice a day, ten repetitions, advancing to multiple sets of ten. If pain continues to the next day, discontinue and discuss with your therapist.

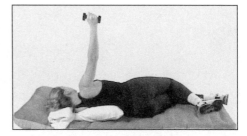

Side-lying arm raises should be done on both sides.

Side-lying external rotation

Lying on your side with the top arm along the edge of your body and with your elbow flexed to ninety degrees, rotate the shoulder in a continuous circular motion. Don't rotate too far, especially if you are hypermobile. Attempt twice a day, ten repetitions, advancing to multiple sets of ten. If pain continues to the next day, discontinue and discuss with your therapist.

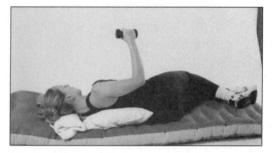

Side-lying external rotation

"Hold up" or prone scapula retraction

Lie prone (face down) with one or two pillows under your chest and a rolled towel under the forehead to allow space for breathing. Position your arms straight out, and bend your

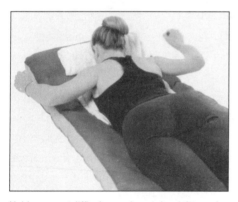

Holdups are a difficult exercise, and weight can be added as tolerated.

elbows to ninety degrees. Now lift your arms off the floor, squeezing the shoulder blades together. Hold this position for three seconds and lower the arms slowly. Attempt to do them twice a day, ten repetitions, advancing to multiple sets of ten. If pain continues to the next day, discontinue and discuss with your therapist.

"V" exercises (Sitting or Standing Shoulder Abduction)

This exercise is best performed in front of a mirror. Sit or stand with both arms close to your body, positioning them slightly forward of your chest. Then bring the extended arms up 35 to 45 degrees while contracting only the deltoids (upper arm muscles).

Try not to activate the upper trapezius (muscles between your neck and shoulder) too soon so that neck soreness is avoided. Attempt to do them twice a day, ten repetitions, advancing to multiple sets of ten. If pain continues to the next day, discontinue and discuss with your therapist.

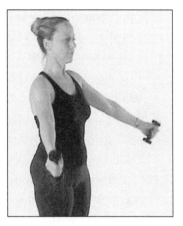

The "V" exercise

Advanced Strengthening Exercises

Advanced exercises can be incorporated into your treatment program after you have mastered the basic five and you feel comfortable with the strengthening program. It is particularly important to perform these exercises under the supervision of your physical or occupational therapist. Progressing through these exercises will strengthen specific muscle groups that are weak and out of balance as a result of RSI. In some cases you may need special equipment more likely to be found in a gym. Again, these exercises should be carried out in sets of ten, advancing to multiple sets of ten.

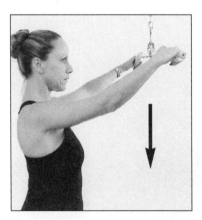

Latissimus dorsi pull-downs are important to develop synchronous shoulder and arm movement as well as strength.

Latissimus dorsi pull-downs

The latissimus dorsi muscle, a large triangular muscle in the back, plays a major role in shoulder and arm movement. It extends, rotates, and moves the arm toward the body and draws the shoulder down and back. Most gyms have a bar attached to a cable and pulley. Face this machine with elbows extended and wrists neutral. Don't grip the bar tightly, and pull down, feeling both latissimus dorsi and abdominal contractions.

Wall push-ups

This exercise stretches, strengthens, and mobilizes front and back upper body muscles. By loosening these tight muscles, pressure is taken off the nerves and blood vessels supplying the arms and hands. Stand, placing your arms above your head and maintaining straight wrists, with your feet a bit out from the wall. Bend your elbows as your chest leans into the wall. This exercise also can be done in a corner.

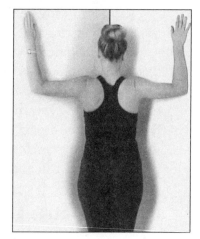

Wall push-ups stretch, strengthen, and mobilize front and back upper body muscles.

Abdominal exercises

These exercises are important for muscle balance and posture. RSI patients should avoid lifting the head off the floor because it irritates the cervical spine. Do this lying down, with your back flat on the floor. Bend the knees, and alternate toe tapping from one foot to the other.

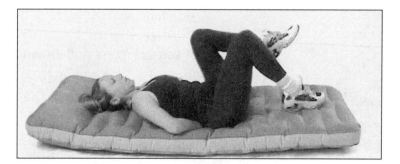

Abdominal exercises are necessary for developing muscle balance and power. These are a critical component of lower back strengthening.

Wrist curls

These exercises will strengthen forearm extension and flexion. They should only be started when stretching and basic exercises have eliminated pain. Weights should start at one pound or less, reaching a maximum of four pounds for the forearm flexors and three pounds for the extensors.

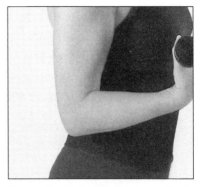

Wrist curls will strengthen forearms. Don't use weights until stretching and basic exercises have eliminated pain.

Supinator pronator exercises

I have found these exercises useful for those with golfer's or tennis elbows. By stretching and strengthening these muscles, pressure is taken off the insertion of the muscles into bone at the elbow. A hammer can be used for this exercise. Start by holding it closest to the hammer's head; work down the handle as you progress. With the elbow at your side flexed to ninety degrees, a two-pound weight is rotated back and forth, working both supinator and pronator muscles.

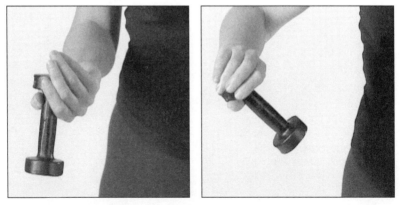

Supinator curl   Pronator curl

Supinator and pronator curls stretch and strengthen forearms and help to relieve medial and lateral epicondylitis. Weight should be added as tolerated. Elbow should be flexed to ninety degrees.

Shoulder shrugs

As an advanced exercise, begin with two-pound weights in each hand and progress according to the recommendation of your therapist.

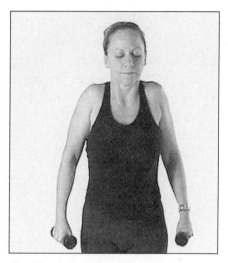

Shoulder shrugs help to loosen tightened shoulder muscles.

Hand intrinsics with putty

The intrinsic muscles of the hand tend to weaken as a result of compromised nerve supply. Using various grades of a special soft putty can strengthen them. Opposing each finger to the thumb, one at a time, squeeze the putty between the finger and the thumb. Do the same between each finger and the adjacent finger in a scissorslike motion. Do ten repetitions per finger.

Different colors of a special putty provide variable resistance.

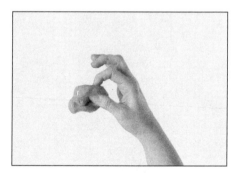

Many other exercises can be incorporated into your treatment program by your therapist that will relate to your particular injuries and your progress.

Manual Therapy: Soft-Tissue Work for RSI

Your therapist may use the terms soft tissue work, manual therapy, or myofascial release. By whatever name, this is the technique that therapists use to mobilize particularly tight muscles in the early stages of RSI treatment, when it is difficult for you to mobilize your soft tissues so you can do your exercises properly. Manual therapy is an important and helpful adjunct to both physical and occupational therapy. Not all therapists are skilled in manual therapy techniques.

The purpose of myofascial release is to locate tightened muscle groups that impinge on nerves, diminish circulation, and restrict mobility. In RSI it involves several levels of activity, which consist of passive stretching by placing thumb or hand pressure on muscles and tendons to produce tension. By applying tension, the therapist passively stretches muscle that, if you attempted to actively stretch yourself, would place too much pressure on the tendons and joints. Active limb movement is the other part of soft-tissue work. While the therapist maintains pressure near these tight areas, the patient actively moves the muscles involved.

For RSI patients, the areas that most commonly benefit from manual therapy include the muscles of the palm, forearm, pectoralis minor and major, scalene, upper trapezius, subscapularis, latissimus dorsi, and scapula. There are also many painful trigger points in the upper and lower back that might need manual therapy.*

---

*Many of the therapies and exercises proposed in this section were developed in conjunction with Lisa Sattler, M.S., P.T., a physical therapist who specializes in the treatment of RSI.

Other Treatment Techniques

There are adjuvant therapies that can be helpful but that should not be your principal treatment for RSI. These include:

Yoga

Yoga can be used as a relaxation technique and is good for channeling stress. Obviously you want to stick to beginner-level positions and avoid any pose that will strain the damaged muscles of your body.

Alexander Technique

F. M. Alexander (1869–1955) was an Australian actor who developed laryngitis while performing. He observed himself while speaking and noted that muscular tension was related to his problem. The technique teaches you to use your muscles appropriately, with the proper amount of exertion for each task. The Alexander technique is useful if there is intrinsic muscle balance and an equality of muscle strength. Therefore, physical therapy and strengthening exercises must be at a level of competence to allow you to benefit from the Alexander technique. You cannot balance your body without strength.

Feldenkrais Method

This method is named after its originator, Dr. Moshe Feldenkrais (1904–1984), a Russian-born physicist, judo expert, mechanical engineer, and educator. The Feldenkrais method is essentially based on physics and biomechanics. It attempts to expand self-image through movement sequences. As in the Alexander technique, it should not be a primary therapy.

Rolfing

This is named after Dr. Ida P. Rolf, who started her work more than fifty years ago. Her program is based on a holistic system of movement education coupled with soft-tissue manipulation. The goal is to make more efficient use of muscles, conserve energy, relieve stress, and diminish pain.

Hellerwork

Hellerwork is named after its originator, Joseph Heller. It is a system of somatic education and structural bodywork based on the inseparability of body, mind, and spirit. It is presented as an eleven-session series whose goal is to release muscle and connective tissue, using deep tissue bodywork techniques. It is based on the assumption that all people are innately healthy.

8

Ergonomics: Making Your Equipment Fit

It is unlikely that ergonomics will become redundant in the office of the information age. In general, experience has shown that with increasing productivity the intensity of human work increases. The load on the sensory organs and mental functions, environmental problems and constrained postures are likely to remain challenges for ergonomics in the future, too.

–Étienne Grandjean, *Ergonomics in Computerized Offices,* 1987

Would you intentionally buy a suit that doesn't fit or run a marathon in one-size-fits-all shoes? Ergonomics is the science of making sure that things fit–that tools, keyboards, musical instruments, and a host of things we use in our daily lives don't harm us.

Dr. Carl Zenz, a professor of medicine at the Medical College of Wisconsin, defines ergonomics as a combination of three things: engineering and physical sciences, behavioral sciences, and biological sciences. Here we look at the engineering and physical sciences part of ergonomics so you can view your work setup from a new perspective.

Ergonomics at the Worksite

Ergonomics *should* be the responsibility of a specialist trained to choose and fit equipment so that each employee gets the right equipment and the right training to use that equipment. A major role for the ergonomist is to keep up with new developments in safety and design and to advise the employer when equipment becomes obsolete or dangerous or when employees are experiencing difficulty or injury at work.

If there is no staff ergonomist, or if you work at home, making the choice of good equipment becomes your job. New chairs, desks, trays, keyboards, input devices such as the mouse, track ball, joystick, and touch pad come on to the market every day. You need a basic understanding of how these products are supposed to function and what features you should look for.

Fitting equipment is important for a number of reasons. First, it is essential to place your body in correct balance to do your work. Just improving ergonomics can begin to reverse the discomfort and pain of RSI. A good workstation setup fosters good posture, which starts you on the road to recovery. Although your body is flexible and adaptable, there is no reason why it should be contorted to fit a chair or a computer setup. Your workstation should be fitted so your body is not subjected to strain and injury.

A well-thought-out ergonomic item should be adaptable to its user. A keyboard as well as a chair must be easily adjustable. Be critical when purchasing ergonomic equipment, as it may be ergonomic in name only. Thousands of products are on the market making claims ranging from curing carpal tunnel syndrome to solving all of your RSI problems, potential or actual. Make your purchase based solely on your need for a more healthful work space, and do it as an informed consumer. Many products such as wrist rests, splints, and other advertised self-treatment devices may be useless and in some cases even harmful. Remember that the best ergonomically designed workstation is useless to you if have bad technique or are in poor physical condition.

Chairs

When evaluating a workstation, I look at seating first and build the rest of the workstation around an ergonomically sound and comfortable chair. A good chair can do much to help your posture. The chair should be soft upholstered but not very soft and should have casters so you can move freely. Recently, chairs with flexible netting have become popular. One consideration is size. A few of the high-end manufacturers make their chairs in different sizes, although most chairs are of the one-size-fits-all variety.

When selecting the chair, make sure that the seat pan supports you comfortably without your buttocks draping over the edges. The seat pan should not be so long that it digs into the back of your thighs, and its front should have a downward-rolled edge. The seat pan should ideally be adjustable so it can tilt to allow the knees to be lower than the hips. Many chairs do not have seat pan tilt, as it requires that the seat pan be separated from the chair's back. If seat pan tilt is not available, a wedge-shaped pillow can be placed on the seat. It is this tilt that carries some of the body weight to the feet and stabilizes the lower spine. Having a seat pan that can slide backward and forward is also desirable.

High-Backed Chairs

Avoid high-backed "executive" chairs if your work involves heavy keyboard use. These chairs, while imposing, tend to lock you in place and prevent free movement of the shoulder blades, which is essential for shoulder and arm mobility. Chair backs should be low enough to allow free shoulder movement.

Armrests

Avoid armrests entirely unless they can be moved out of the way while working. Leaning on them while keying prevents you from using the shoulder and upper back muscles, making your forearms and hands do all the work. If you need armrests, they should be the stubby kind, so you can't lean on them when you type and they won't bump into the desk.

Easy Adjustability

My patients have complained about chairs with multiple levers that are difficult to operate with their injuries. Look for a chair that has a simple mechanism. Adjust the chair properly for computer work, and sit in it for a few minutes before you buy it.

Kneeling Chairs

Some people prefer backless kneeler chairs, made popular in Scandinavian countries. They can place pressure on the knee joints and should be used with caution. If you use a kneeling chair, alternate it with a traditional chair while you work to distribute the muscle load of your body.

Standing

For those who are comfortable keying while standing or who have to stand, as at an airlines reservation counter, the height of your keyboard is important. Whenever you work without a neutral wrist position you are endangering your upper body. If your wrists are bent upward, as if you are pushing open a door, you must change the height or the angle of the keyboard to prevent injury. Keyboard users who stand tend to flex their elbows tightly, causing tension of the ulnar nerve at the elbow. They are also more at risk for low back problems.

Footrests

Avoid angled footrests unless they are fixed in place. If you need one, it is better to have a footrest that keeps your foot flat, though above the ground. The footrest should be big enough to move your feet around without falling off the edges. No foot-dangling. If your legs are too short to reach the floor, get the right footrest.

Desks

When manual typewriters were the standard, office desks often had two levels: the standard desk height, about twenty-eight or twenty-nine inches high, and the "return," about twenty-six inches high, where the typewriter was placed. This would place the desk at the right height for writing and put the typewriter in a comfortable position for manual typing. The chair would swivel into either position for work. This configuration has largely disappeared from the office.

A standard desk height is appropriate for writing and sorting papers but is usually too high for keyboard placement. By placing the keyboard at desk height and resting your forearms on the desktop, you get no help from the strong muscles of the shoulders or the upper back. If your keyboard is at desk height, you are reaching too high, clearly a recipe for trouble. Those desks that come with a special keyboard pullout drawer that is in a fixed, flat position and cannot be tilted, also are troublesome. Since the height of most desks is fixed, adjustable pullout trays can overcome some of the height problems.

Your desktop probably has a phone setup. Be sure you have it placed where your hand can easily reach it and that you have a headset jack on it. If you use the phone a lot while you use the computer, a headset should be on your head! Never cradle the telephone on your shoulder, and absolutely never when you are using the computer. Cradling the phone is so injurious that you should invest in your own headset if you can't get your employer to supply you with one.

Pullout Trays

If you are doing more than one or two hours of keyboard work at a time, a pullout tray with an adjustable negative tilt capability as illustrated on the next page, is a good solution. These can usually be attached to the underside of a desk or table. The tray should be height-adjustable and should have negative tilt capability—that is, you should be able to tilt it away from you, and

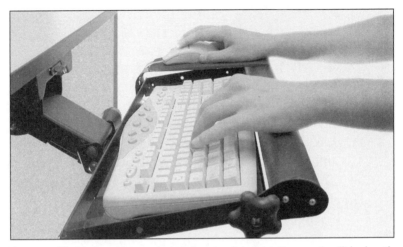

Figure 20. The ideal position, particularly for a touch typist, is the negative tilt keyboard tray as shown. Note the neutral wrist position.

not just pull it out flat. A half-inch block or shim under the near end of your keyboard will give a negative tilt if your flat pullout tray is low enough to keep your wrists in a neutral position. The tilt makes the keys harder to see, so negative tilt trays work better for touch typists than for those who hunt and peck. The tray should be large enough to accommodate a standard or split keyboard, with some space available for an input device such as a mouse, track ball, or touch pad. Make sure your knees clear the hinge attachment, since a central hinge can obstruct knee movement.

Some trays have an extra fixed or sliding mouse bridge that can be placed over the number keys. This feature is desirable, since it keeps your hands and arms comfortably close in to the keyboard. If you are not a touch typist, the pullout tray may be difficult for you, and you may be forced to keep it flat.

Computer Keyboards

No other piece of computer equipment has had more design research and gone through more style changes than the computer keyboard. Research has focused on key placement, size, adjustability, touch, key pressure, and technical design. Still, the keyboard that suits everyone has not yet appeared.

What kind of keyboard should you buy? Choosing a keyboard can be confusing, as there are so many available at a wide range of prices. When you buy a new computer, it comes with a standard keyboard, and if it is not comfortable or is causing you pain, you will want to get one that suits your needs better. As mentioned in chapter 2, the elbow carrying angle, which varies from person to person, will affect the way you place your hands as you hit the keys. The greater your carrying angle, the greater the likelihood that you will need a split keyboard. In any case, I believe a split keyboard is generally a good choice for everyone.

Virtually all keyboards now on the market have the cheaper-to-manufacture membrane cushioning for keys, rather than the more desirable individual spring loading for each key, which is best for good touch feedback. Basically, three types of keyboards are available: traditional, fixed split, and adjustable split. The traditional keyboard is supplied with most home computers and is usually what you will find at your workstation. Some are available with a number pad on the right side, while others are alphanumeric or have a separate number keyboard.

The fixed split keyboard has a split at an angle of about twenty-four degrees and a slight downward taper on each end, which takes the hand slightly out of the palms-down position.

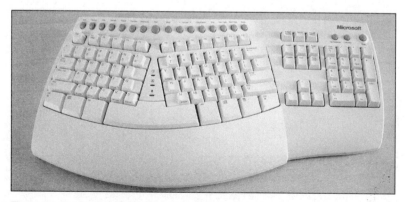

Figure 21. The fixed split keyboard is ideal for most people.

The number pad, on the right side, is flat. The palm apron along the front edge of these keyboards is not ergonomically sound—don't rely on it to support your palms. Small legs that prop up the far end of the keyboard should not be used, since they encourage extending your wrist, as when pushing a door open, a harmful posture. If you purchase this type of keyboard, make sure you have the right size of pullout tray.

There are several varieties of adjustable keyboards. These keyboards can be placed in the traditional position, angled, and even tented so the hands are no longer in the palms-down position but are held somewhere between palms up and palms down.

According to Dr. Alan Hedge, an ergonomics researcher at Cornell University, keying with the palms in a vertical position, as in playing an accordion, allows the forearm tendons, which move the fingers, to work more easily. Since you cannot see the keys in this position, it is difficult or impossible for a nontouch typist to use one, so vertical mirrors are installed on each side. Many of the people who feel uncomfortable in the palms-down position at the keyboard have tight forearm pronator and supinator muscles, which need to be stretched. By placing the adjustable keyboard at a tented angle of approximately thirty degrees they might feel more comfortable during their retraining. See chapter 6 for details on exercises.

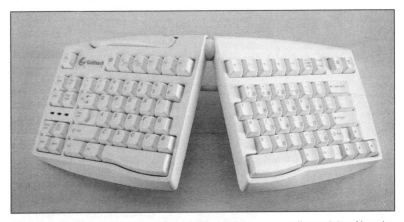

Figure 22. The adjustable keyboard is suitable for daily use as well as training. Note the split spacebar.

Hot Keys

Many keyboards have hot keys, which can cut down on repetitive activities. They are especially useful for persons at risk for RSI because they diminish the workload. You can have a hot key for Internet availability; e-mail; multimedia; sleep; and custom hot keys that you can program. Some keyboards also have labels for CTRL key shortcuts. More of these options are available for PC users than for Mac users.

Touch and Tactile Feedback

Dr. David Rempel at UCLA and Dr. Thomas Armstrong at the University of Michigan have done extensive research on the amount of work spent in activating keys. Basically, this research has shown that most of us press the keys with far greater force than we need to. Most keyboards no longer have spring-loaded keys, which are more costly to manufacture. Now a plastic or rubber membrane cushions the keys, so that the sense of contact is lost, as is the "click" that told you that you made contact. The effort required to be sure you've struck the key increases your workload and potential for injury.

Wrist Rests

The use of wrist rests is controversial. I prefer to call them wrist guides and ask my patients to use them only as guides, because resting the forearms on a wrist support while keying can be harmful for several reasons. First, they take the upper arms out of the process of keying, so you are overloading the forearm and hand muscles and increasing your chances of injury. Moreover, the wrist support tends to encourage potentially harmful positioning, particularly wrist extension (bending your wrist up, as in pushing a door open). With the wrist fixed on the wrist rest, there is a tendency to use a windshield-wiperlike wrist motion, which is extra work and harmful. Finally, the wrist rest places pressure over the carpal tunnel area, which is not a good idea.

Movable cradles that attach to the desk to support your forearms, or chair arms that allow keying while you rest your arms on the chair are potentially just as harmful.

The Virtual Keyboard

Some day you may be able to sit at a desk with a small projection device in front of you and type on a projected keyboard. According to an article in the *Scientific American* of January 2003, a pair of inventors came up with a concept of remote control for electronic devices. This virtual keyboard called the Canesta Keyboard Perception Chipset consists of three parts. To quote the article:

"The device consists of a pattern projector, an infrared light source and a sensor. The pattern projector uses a small laser only 9 millimeters on each side to produce what looks like an ordinary keyboard on a desk." According to the first users of this system, they found the lack of tactile feedback a problem, so a click was added. It may take some time for people to get used to this way of typing, which experienced typists at first found somewhat slower than a standard keyboard, although practice may produce additional speed. The device offers the potential for easily placing a keyboard in a comfortable position in almost any work environment.

Laptop Computers

Laptop computers are now very popular in businesses, schools, and homes. Thousands of students are taking laptops to class, using them to take notes and look up data. Laptops have a number of ergonomic disadvantages. They are small and have a constricted keyboard. They can be heavy when carried or actually used on your lap. The laptop screen is generally not separable from the keyboard, making ergonomic placement difficult. Input devices are miniaturized and difficult to operate. And there is considerable variability in the brightness and clarity of laptop screens.

For picture clarity, your best bet is to try laptops in a store, where they can be compared side by side before buying. Try to rent or borrow one to test it before buying. Special desks for laptops are now on the market; bring your laptop with you to try them out. Always attach a normal keyboard to your laptop when possible and set the screen at the proper height and angle.

Laptops: A Warning

Laptop computers are a great convenience, and the new wireless systems make them even handier. If you have ever used one without a desk support, you may have noticed that they get hot! A Swedish researcher described the case of a fifty-year-old man who placed his laptop computer on his lap and used it for about an hour (*Lancet* 360, no. 9346 [2002]:1704). The heat from the computer was noticeable but not severe, causing a burning sensation in his thighs; the burning sensation disappeared when he repositioned the laptop. The following day he noticed swelling and irritation of his penis, followed by redness and blistering on his scrotum. The blisters, which were manifestations of a second-degree burn, burst and became infected but ultimately healed. The slow burn occurred even though he was fully dressed in trousers and underwear. Needless to say, he was greatly inconvenienced. The laptop computer user should simply remember to keep a pillow or some form of cushioning between the laptop and the lap.

Computer Input Devices

The Mouse

The mouse is a significant source of injury for computer users. These point-and-click devices generally conform to the shape of your hand, are usually right-hand-oriented, and cause you to flex your index or middle fingers to activate the screen arrow. The thumb and opposing fourth and fifth fingers usually grip the mouse. If the grip is too intense, you risk getting thumb and finger tendinitis.

There are great numbers of mice on the market with features that claim to make life easier for the user. Lately optical mice have been introduced, which work on any surface but glass. They seem to require less effort to move the arrow around on the screen. Some mice have multiple functions similar to those of hot keys.

Placement of the mouse is critical. When placed too high and too far to the side, the mouse can cause shoulder and bicep tendinitis as well as muscle fatigue. Ideally, the mouse should be at the same level as the keyboard and as central to the body as practically possible. Hold the mouse as loosely as possible, with little or no gripping.

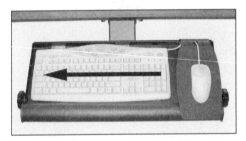

Figure 23. The floating mouse tray allows the mouse to move to a central and more comfortable position.

The Track Ball

This device is frequently used as a replacement for the standard mouse. The track ball comes in different sizes but is generally about the size of a golf ball set into a fixed holder. Smaller rollers can be found on some laptop computers.

There are certain advantages to the track ball. Since you don't need a mouse pad, or a large surface to move around on, you can place the track ball anywhere you want. Moving the ball makes you use your stronger upper arm muscles more. As long as your hand is held slightly cupped and relaxed, the track ball is a good substitute for the mouse.

Don't overextend your fingers flat out over the track ball, because this will work the wrong muscles.

The Touch Pad

The touch pad is operated by running a finger over its surface to move the screen arrow. Like the track ball, you can place it where it is most comfortable. In addition to the standard touch pad, most laptops are now equipped with a small, centrally located touch pad.

Researchers at the University of Michigan have expressed some misgivings about the touch pad based on their findings. I suspect that this is because there is a tendency to use one extended finger to do all the work. If your hand is

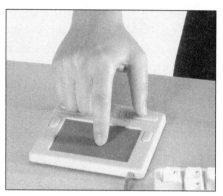

Figure 24. Touchpad showing proper use

relaxed, your fingers are slightly curved, and you alternate the fingers used, then the touch pad can be useful.

Other Input Devices

Wands, pens, joysticks, and other devices are on the market. There are wireless mice that fit on the fingers and work simply by moving the fingers against each other. Tiny joysticks, set among the keys, are used on some laptop computers, although they may be difficult to control. Here you have to be your own judge. There is no reason why you shouldn't alternate among any of the various input devices to minimize the likelihood of injury.

Pens and Pencils

The original "input device" is the pen or pencil, and almost everyone I have seen with RSI has difficulty with them. Holding the pen too tightly is a common problem. To break the tight grip, widen the barrel of the pen by purchasing sponge curlers used to set hair. Remove the plastic holder, then insert the pen through the hole in the middle of the curler. This provides a soft cushion for the fingers and widens the grip.

Although there are also many expensive pens that you can buy with expanded cushioned bands, they are less effective than the curler, which is so cheap you can have one for each of your writing instruments.

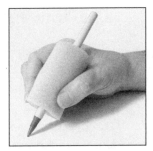

Figure 25. A hair curler with a pen inserted inside can be far more comfortable for writing.

Other Computer-Related Ergonomic Factors

Document Holders

Document holders are particularly helpful if used correctly. They attach to either side of the computer screen and have a clip to hold one or more papers. Always place the document holder on the side of your dominant eye. See chapter 4 for more details.

Monitors

The standard monitor consists of a cathode ray tube (CRT), usually ranging from seventeen to twenty-one inches in size. Companies may sell their own brand along with their computer, or they can be purchased separately. Size is generally based on the diagonal measurement—a 17-inch CRT really has a viewable image size of sixteen inches. If you work with graphics or spreadsheets you'll want a nineteen-inch screen or even a twenty- or twenty-one-inch screen.

Flat-panel liquid crystal displays (LCDs) are becoming more common and take up less room than a standard CRT and weigh considerably less. Flat-panel displays give a very clear image but have a more limited color range. An important consideration and inherent disadvantage is that they are best viewed straight on because contrast is lost as you move off center. Before buying a monitor, try it out in the store. Check to see if text is as clear on the edges as at the center. Do the picture colors look clear and natural? Compare the monitors side by side if you can.

LCD Projectors

LCD projectors attached to computers are usually used at conferences or meetings with presentation software to enlarge the viewing area to a wall or screen. They also can give the visually impaired a chance to work with computers, and in some cases, may enhance a legally blind person's function at the computer. New LCD or plasma TV screens also can be used to obtain a large, comfortable picture.

Voice-Activated Software

Whether you have RSI or not, if you want to use voice recognition equipment, certain rules apply. A few hours of training with a speech therapist may be helpful to teach you how to enunciate properly, avoid slurring words, move smoothly through your dictation, and avoid straining your voice. Using the right microphone and placing it properly controls your speaking quality and volume. Don't forget that voice-activated systems need lots of RAM. Look for Internet Web sites such as http://www. voicerecognition.net for guidance about what to buy—the software is constantly being improved. The experience of one voice-activated-software user (W. Wayne Gibbs, *Scientific American,* June 2002) is worth noting. He calculated that his voice recognition system reduced his mousing by roughly a third in e-mail, by more than half in file management, and by two-thirds in Web surfing.

Changing Workstations

Many people change workstations daily or share them. Carry a tape measure and use it to adjust your workstation so you have consistent work conditions. This applies to the entire workstation, not just your chair measurements. Car manufacturers now provide automatically adjustable "smart" seats to suit several drivers using one car. Someday we may have "smart" chairs and desks for computer users.

Ergonomics and Stress

Recently I came across some fascinating work by Dr. Erik Peper, a professor of holistic health at San Francisco State University. He points out that even if you have the best ergonomic setup possible, just sitting down at your desk can produce physical reactions that can increase stress. In his studies Dr. Peper found that 95 percent of persons raised their shoulders as they sat down at the computer. This observation impressed me because it ties in with the postural problems we see so often in people with RSI. Your ergonomic setup is supposed to get you into a comfortable position, yet sitting down and shrugging your shoulders is the very posture that will place more tension on an important nerve area, the brachial plexus. Dr. Peper also noted that 30 percent of people began shallow breathing as they sat at the computer. He theorizes that computers, for whatever reason, trigger a fight-or-flight response accompanied by an adrenaline rush. Inhaling slowly can trigger the body's relaxation response and help to quiet this reaction. There are many stress reduction techniques that can be very helpful, but the main thing is not to drop your guard by thinking that good equipment alone will protect you from injury.

Can these observations be applied to other activities? Does the musician or the court stenographer raise shoulders or breathe superficially beginning his or her activity? Is this a stress reaction that is contributing to the genesis of injury? It seems to me that more work needs to be done in this area and that Dr. Peper's observations are a good starting point.

An Ergonomic Equipment Checklist

Here is a checklist of factors you should keep in mind as you set up or improve your workstation:

Seating

___ Proper size seat pan for your body

___ Seat pan has downward-rolled front edge

___ Adjustable seat pan tilt

___ Wedge pillow if no pan tilt available

___ Seat pan moves both forward and backward

___ Seat back height adjustable to allow shoulder movement

___ Ease of adjustment

___ Adjustable armrests or no armrests

___ Short armrests that don't bump into desk

___ Adjustable seat height

___ Adjustable backrest tilt

___ Soft seat

___ Movable on casters and swivels

Footrest

___ Flat

___ Angled

Desk

___ Desk height

___ Arrangement of desk equipment

Phone

___ Location

___ Phone jack

___ Phone headset

Pullout Tray

___ Adjustable with negative tilt

___ Knee room

___ Large enough to accommodate keyboard

Keyboard

___ Standard

___ Fixed split

___ Adjustable split

Input Devices

___ Placement

___ Mouse: standard or optical

___ Track ball

___ Touch pad

___ Joystick

___ Other

Monitor

___ CRT or LCD

___ Height

___ Size

___ Distance

___ Location

___ Tilt

___ Antiglare screen or shield

___ Flicker

Document Holder

___ Located closer to dominant eye

Writing Tools

___ Ergonomic pen or expander

Where Are We Heading in Ergonomics?

In 1999, the Department of Labor through its Occupational Safety and Health Administration (OSHA) proposed a series of workplace standards. The objective of these standards (29CFR Part 1910) was to address the significant risk of work-related musculoskeletal disorders confronting workers in various jobs. General industry employers covered by the standard would be required to establish an ergonomic program containing some or all of the elements typical of a successful ergonomics program as outlined here:

- Management leadership and employee participation
- Job hazard analysis and control
- Hazard information and reporting
- Training
- Work injury management
- Program evaluation

Under the second Bush administration, the standards rapidly fell victim to House and Senate rejection, despite the many years in preparation, partly because they were thought costly and onerous to businesses, and partly because the standards were cumbersome and confusing. Nevertheless, some state laws preserve these or similar standards.

The proposed federal standards would have affected approximately 1.9 million employers and 27.3 million employees. OSHA estimated that the standards would prevent about 3 million work-related injuries over the following ten years.

9

Biomechanics: Using Your Body

Our body is a machine for living. It is organized for that, it is its nature.

–Leo Tolstoy (1828–1910), *War and Peace*

Our focus, in biomechanics, is how we interact with our tools and how we can do so without incurring injury. There is an important relationship between ergonomics, the external factor or equipment, and biomechanics, the internal factor or the body. The essence of this relationship is that optimal biomechanical activity is easiest to achieve if the groundwork has been laid by using ergonomically sound equipment. If you are not physically and mentally fit and your workstation is not adequately set up, you can't expect to be able to use the equipment without injuring yourself, no matter how much you know about proper technique. Biomechanical training or retraining is the critical final step in a program that will help you recover from RSI.

The Importance of Training and Retraining

Musicians are taught technique, which is a form of biomechanical training, as well as the basic elements of music. Unfortunately, most music teachers have little or no background in the biomechanical or ergonomic aspects of musicianship and rely on what tradition has taught them. The same is true for training to use the computer, where emphasis is on learning to use software and not how to set up a workstation ergonomically and use your body in a biomechanically sound fashion.

A Personal Issue

Each of us has uniquely different physical characteristics. Some of us have long arms or fingers. Some are double-jointed. Some are tall, others short. The variations are infinite. No two persons position themselves at a workstation in the same way. They move their bodies in ways that are subtly, and sometimes not so subtly, different.

Equipment used must fit the user properly, so that you can move in a biomechanically safe way. Biomechanics is a personal issue—a cookbook approach is not acceptable. A five-foot, two-inch woman and a six-foot man cannot share equipment that is not adjusted for each of them.

A Dynamic Process

You can observe your movements, but you are likely to miss many of the subtleties of potential injurious moves and postures with the naked eye. Using videotape to document movement is a very useful way of studying work habits.

I routinely videotape my patients at work or in a simulated work setup. Time-lapse or real-time videotaping shows us what we are doing with our bodies. Both the trainer and the subject can study and correct awkward movements and positioning. With video evaluation, what had formerly been a matter of experience and a trained eye has become a partnership with the patient. People are usually surprised when they see how poorly they perform their work tasks. Try having someone videotape you at your workstation and see what I mean.

Occupational physicians at the University of Connecticut Occupational Health Service, where I am a consultant, are also developing new techniques, such as infrared videotaping, as diagnostic tools. This technique could reveal abnormal movements that need attention and set standards of movement.

Workstation Biomechanics

Posture

When your mother told you to sit up straight, she was right! Throughout this book we have emphasized the importance of good posture. Good posture is best achieved by correcting muscle imbalances. This includes stretching and strengthening muscles that have either sagged or tightened, and thereby developing muscular balance among the neck, upper back, and chest. Even breathing can be affected because of tightened muscles that restrict rib cage movement.

Good posture is also helped by sitting in an easily adjustable chair, positioning the keyboard and the monitor comfortably, and having appropriate, specially corrected computer eyeglasses when necessary. Be sure that you have your telephone placed where your hand can easily reach it, and if you use the phone a lot while you use the computer, a headset should be on your head. Never cradle the telephone on your shoulder. See chapters 4 and 7 for more on this.

The postural deficiencies most often seen among computer users include rounded shoulders and a head thrust forward combined with shoulders that lack free range of motion. Postural deterioration evolves over time in those who don't make efforts to prevent it from occurring. Exercises to maintain or improve posture are detailed in chapter 7.

Wearing a heavy backpack can damage your posture. For years, hikers and outdoor people have used backpacks to carry heavy loads of equipment, and now people are replacing handbags, briefcases, and schoolbags with backpacks. When used indiscriminately, backpacks can lead to postural misalignment. A particularly vulnerable group is young students, as we will see later in this chapter.

Correcting your postural deficiencies is one of the most important things you can do, but it is hard to do without the guidance of an occupational or physical therapist.

Positioning Yourself at the Computer

Dorsiflexion or Wrist Extension

Look carefully at figure 26 and notice this common but extremely harmful position. Compare it with figure 27.

Usually dorsiflexion happens when the keyboard is placed on a desk with the arms resting on the desk surface, which normally is too high for proper keying. In an attempt to do some-

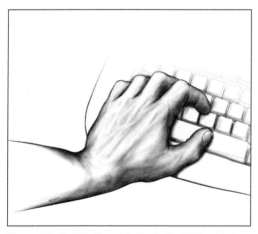

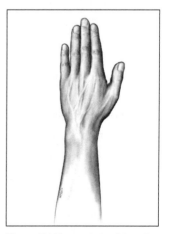

Figure 26. The dorsiflexed (extended) wrist is a biomechanically harmful position.

Figure 27. The neutral wrist position is biomechanically efficient.

thing ergonomic, many manufacturers have placed small, retractable legs at the far end of the keyboard—the wrong end! Using these makes matters worse by increasing the angle of the extended wrist as you key. I haven't been able to figure out why these legs are placed there except perhaps as an attempt to imitate the step up of the mechanical typewriter.

The old typewriters, however, made it impossible to hit the keys with your wrists and forearms on the desk, which forced you to keep a neutral and correct position while typing. There are clear reasons why dorsiflexion is harmful. First, with the wrist extended, one set of forearm muscles (the flexors) is stretched, while another (the extensors) is shortened. The shortened muscles have to pull against the stronger set of flexor muscles to keep the wrist in an extended position (static loading), causing fatigue from overuse. Static loading occurs when the muscle appears to be still, although it actually is working with the added disadvantage of decreased blood supply.

The extended wrist position also involves the flexor muscle group of the forearm in a detrimental way. The flexors are working to press the computer keys in a stretched state. This is an example of eccentric muscle contraction. It is like pulling on an already stretched rubber band, which is the most harmful way a muscle can be used.

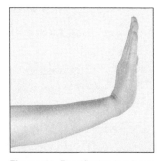

Figure 28. Dorsiflexion is a harmful posture for computer users.

It is very important to keep the wrist in a straight line (neutral position) so that tendons and other soft-tissue structures glide in a more or less straight direction. This is sometimes more easily achieved if an under-the-desktop pullout tray for your keyboard is used and put into a downward slope away from your body.

This position has an added advantage since it takes the elbow beyond the ninety-degree right angle that we so often see in ergonomic pictures. This right-angle position is incorrect because it places more pull on the ulnar nerve at the elbow.

If you are not a touch typist and feel you must keep your arms on the desk surface, make sure your chair is adjusted high enough so you can maintain a neutral wrist position and the shoulders feel comfortable. In any case, make sure you keep your feet firmly on the floor or on a raised platform if your feet don't reach the floor. As you key and use the mouse or other input device, move your entire arm from the shoulder, instead of just activating the wrist.

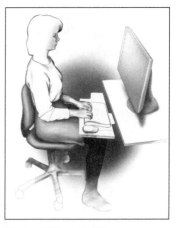

Figure 29. Seated at the computer. Wrists in a straight line, elbows slightly open past ninety degrees, good lower back support, feet on the floor, seat pan tilted downward, keyboard tray tilted downward, mouse close by

Ulnar and radial deviation (windshield wiper wrists)

The next most common harmful position is ulnar and radial deviation.

This position subjects the forearm tendons to twist and kink as they move the fingers. The consequences are strained and inflamed tendons, including lateral epicondylitis, DeQuervain's tenosynovitis, and overworked muscles.

Try to avoid the outer positions you see in figure 30, where the hands move like a pair of windshield wipers. From a biomechanical standpoint, these movements happen for a number of reasons. The most common is limited shoulder use, where placing the forearms on the desk surface restricts the large muscles of the shoulder from moving the arm. This is common in people who key, use a mouse, or play on a musical keyboard. The tendon kinking that results from ulnar and radial deviation probably also contributes to carpal tunnel syndrome, by increasing

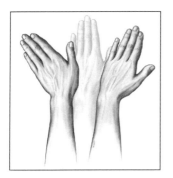

Figure 30 (left to right). Radial Deviation, Neutral, Ulnar Deviation

friction and causing swelling and inflammation within the closed space of the carpal tunnel. Some of the new keyboards now available are angled to reduce the tendency to place the wrists in ulnar deviation. Other keyboards may have a central adjustment, which enables the angle of the keyboard to vary.

The Carrying Angle at the Elbow

Another factor that contributes to increasing the likelihood of ulnar and radial deviation relates to the carrying angle at the elbow. We are all born with different carrying angles of a fixed angle for each person between the humerus and the ulnar bones. Among my patients, this angle is usually 5 to 10 degrees for males. Women normally have a greater angle, usually 10 to 15 degrees.

Compare figure 31 where the subject has a low angle, with figure 32, where the subject has an increased angle. In figure 33

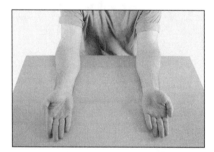

Figure 31. This person has low carrying angle at the elbow.

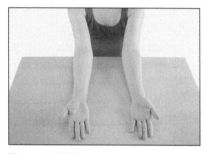

Figure 32. This person has an increased carrying angle at the elbow. Compare with figure 31.

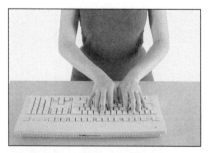

Figure 33. People with an increased carrying angle tend to go into ulnar deviation at the standard keyboard.

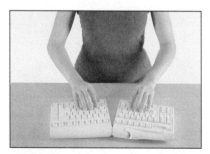

Figure 34. Correction of the patient seen in Figure 33 uses a split keyboard, resulting in a neutral wrist position.

note the subject with hands in pronation placed on the standard keyboard, and also note the resulting ulnar deviation, which is corrected by splitting the keyboard, in figure 34. I recommend a split keyboard for persons with a carrying angle greater than 10 degrees.

If you are overweight, your own body presents an obstacle to placing your arms against your sides. Flexed arms are pronated farther apart by the obese typist, who is forced to go into ulnar deviation.

Finger hyperextension

Another common but harmful keyboard technique is finger hyperextension, which means that instead of maintaining curved fingers (so that you can't see your fingernails), the fingers are extended flat on the keyboard. People with short fingers often get into trouble, straining to reach a distant key. This straining is often the cause of pain in the forearm and elbow,

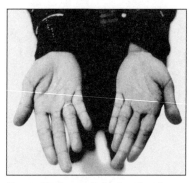

Figure 35. Congenitally short fourth and fifth fingers may be obstacles to comfortable keying or playing certain musical instruments.

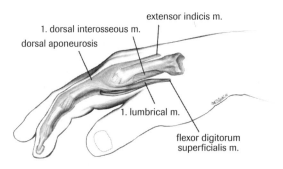

Figure 36. Muscles controlling finger movements. Intrinsics: lumbricals and interossei; extrinsics: extensor indicis and flexor digitorum superficialis. The rounded area at the knuckle is where the dorsal hood is located.

which mystifies the examining physician or therapist because the connection between the short fingers and the biomechanics at the keyboard is not recognized.

Women with long nails are more or less forced into hyperextension. Get rid of long nails, because they force you to hit the keys with fingers extended. The maximum nail length for a typist should be $\frac{1}{16}$ inch.

If we study the function of the hand, we see why hyperextension (holding the fingers completely flat out) is harmful. This concept is often poorly understood because it involves knowing that the intrinsic muscles of the hand can have dual functions. The muscles involved are called lumbricals and interossei (see figure 36). The main function of the lumbricals is to flex the fingers downward from the knuckle joints to the tips of the fingers. The main function of the interossei is to spread the fingers apart and pull them together. In the case of the lumbricals, they help the forearm flexor muscles to flex the fingers. In hyperextension, however, both the lumbricals and the interossei act as finger extensors, which means that they are lost as flexors. We have not only lost the intrinsic hand muscles as flexors, to help us hit the keyboard, but as extensors, they now work against the forearm flexor muscles as the extended fingers try to hit the keys.

Try to flex your fingers while they are in extension and see how much harder it is! Curve your fingers slightly and you will have maximum finger mobility. It is important especially for pianists to understand this concept.

Finger hyperflexion

If the fingers are overflexed (hyperflexion), as in a fist position, they cannot spread apart but can be pulled together. Try this by attempting to spread your fingers while making a fist. The fingers can only be fully spread while they are extended (hyperextension). Hyperextension and hyperflexion are extremes that are inefficient for hand use. Between these two extreme hand positions is a middle ground where the hand operates efficiently and safely.

Alienated or hyperextended thumb

In observing many people typing, especially those who touch-type, I have found a significant percentage who are using only one thumb to press the space bar. The unused thumb is constantly held up and outward, alienating it from the rest of the typing fingers. Try holding one thumb in this position and you will see that the fingers tend to hyperextend, making it more difficult to flex them and placing greater strain on both hand and forearm muscles. This causes loss of dexterity and efficiency and can lead to tendinitis at the base of the thumb. The group action of the thumb and fingers is complex. To retrain yourself it may be necessary, at least temporarily, to eliminate both thumbs from keyboarding, which will slow your typing speed until you heal. Normally, the faster you type the more likely you are to get injured.

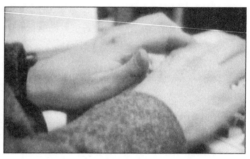

Figure 37. An alienated thumb, held away from the spacebar. This is an inefficient use of hand muscles.

Thumb hyperflexion

Moving the thumb downward and tucking it under the palm is commonly seen among musicians doing arpeggios and occasionally among typists. This repetitive thumb hyperflexion can cause DeQuervain's tenosynovitis.

Unusual Biomechanical Actions

Kneading

Some keyboard users continually flex and extend their fingers while at the keyboard in a dough-kneading action. This is an inefficient movement that increases their workload substantially and predisposes them to greater likelihood of injury.

Clacking

Clackers hit the keys much harder than necessary. Only slight pressure is necessary to activate computer keys, yet many people pound so hard that one can hear them from far off. This technique aberration can be a sign of stress or simply a bad habit. It literally adds tons of pressure that you need not exert. Certain of my patients who have complained of fingertip pain or numbness when examined, turn out to be clackers. They may also be at risk for developing vibration syndrome. So lighten up! Practice lighter touch by gradually teaching yourself to control the force of the stroke.

Incorrect mouse use

Another source of thumb tendinitis is the mouse. Although mouse placement is critical to prevent arm and shoulder problems, it is the gripping of the mouse that leads to a disabling thumb tendinitis. Having the mouse higher than the keyboard (flexion) or too far to the side (ulnar or radial deviation) or using it with the wrist bent up (extension) are all awkward positions that need to be corrected with biomechanical retraining. Some typists stretch their fingers flat out while using the mouse, the touch pad, or a track ball, which is very inefficient because it pits the flexor muscles against the extensors.

RSI and Kids

Backpacks carried by the current generation of students have become mobile lockers. The average student carries a backpack that can weigh twenty pounds or more, and orthopedists are reporting more and more children with back pain. A recent study by the American Academy of Orthopedic Surgeons reported that 58 percent of orthopedists saw children complaining of back and shoulder pain caused by these heavy backpacks.

These are the same students who are likely to spend many hours at computer keyboards and as they grow older become more and more at risk for the type of postural-related injury we discuss in this book. The American Academy of Orthopedic Surgeons recommends that a backpack should not exceed 20 percent of a child's body weight. If you are feeling pain, try avoiding backpack use for two weeks; if the pain subsides, then the cause is probably the backpack. First, try to eliminate all unnecessary books. For any backpack user, an upper body exercise program should be part of the daily routine. Kids might not think they're cool, but backpacks on wheels are now available and should be considered.

By the time growth ceases—usually between fourteen and seventeen—children become more susceptible to injury. This is especially true for young musicians and athletes. There are several reasons for this. Soft tissues that were once extremely pliable begin to assume an adult configuration, and postural characteristics begin to solidify. Growth hormone levels diminish, resulting in a decreased capacity for muscle regeneration. A body once capable of overcoming biomechanical and ergonomic deficiencies becomes more susceptible to injury. Without early education and prevention, the risk of injury increases.

Schools, Posture, and Computers

Researchers at Cornell University have confirmed my own observation that many of the elementary school computer labs are not set up with healthy typing posture in mind. A 1999 study of schools by Shawn Oates appeared in the journal *Computers in the Schools* and found "striking misfits" between children and computer workstations. Typically, keyboards and monitors were placed too high. Hunched shoulders, awkward wrist positions, and hyperextended necks were some of the findings.

My own observations suggest that this situation also exists in the classrooms and libraries of colleges and universities. Graduate students working long hours on their theses seem particularly susceptible. Another less obvious area is the home, where young students use computers set up for their parents.

"Yips" in Golfers

Sports can not only contribute to symptoms of RSI, but also can be affected by it. This is especially true where precision of movement is required. An article in the *Wall Street Journal* of February 19, 2003, described a curious condition that golfers call "yips." A golfer with yips would notice spasmodic jerking as he or she crouched over a putt, often causing the golfer to miss. The condition has been studied at the Mayo Clinic, where a definitive conclusion as to its origin has not been reached. No one is sure whether the condition is physical, mental, or both. Some suggest it may be a form of focal dystonia (see chapter 13).

I have seen several golfers with similar symptoms. These were recreational golfers who worked in fields requiring computer use. In these patients, I found postural problems and other troubles, including neurogenic thoracic outlet. I instructed them to bring their clubs to the next visit so we could videotape their actions. The results were revealing. While putting, their shoulders were rounded and their heads were thrust forward, a position that can compress the nerves of the brachial plexus between two scalene muscles of the neck. The golf swing put traction and compression on these same nerves.

In my limited experience, "yips" was not much different from other RSI cases where posture plays a role in compromising the function of the muscles in the arms, forearms, and hands because of brachial plexus injury. The role of stress and resulting psychological problems have been suggested as factors contributing to "yips." The few golfers I have seen did improve with a regimen of physical therapy, home exercises, and psychological counseling. Anyone presenting with "yips" symptoms should be thoroughly examined to obtain a diagnosis, just like anyone who presents with symptoms of RSI and its complications.

10

At Home
with RSI

Mid pleasures and palaces though we may roam
Be it ever so humble, there's no place like home.

–J. H. Payne (1791–1852)

The term "activities of daily living" applies to the ordinary things you do every day—using the computer, driving, talking on the phone, reading a book or newspaper, brushing your teeth, cooking, gardening, opening doors, turning faucet knobs, and hundreds of others. Normally, we perform these functions easily, without noticing we are doing them. For someone suffering from RSI, these tasks may become a huge burden because of pain and weakness. These physical shortcomings can be heightened by a sense of frustration, helplessness, anxiety, panic, and depression. Some of these day-to-day tasks can be made easier by doing things differently and using tools that can help.

When you are recovering from RSI, improvement in the ability to perform tasks is an important sign that you are getting better. During your initial physical evaluation, discussing your limitations in activities of daily living can aid in the diagnosis of your illness. These functional limits give your physician and therapists information about what activities may be contributing to your injury outside of work.

The following suggestions come from a variety of sources, including patients, therapists, and health and safety committees. Lisa Sattler M.S., P.T., a physical therapist who specializes in treating patients with RSI (she has a Web site at http://www. lisasattler.com), and Vera Wills, a musicians' ergonomist, have also been extremely helpful in providing me with information derived from their own experience.

Most people with RSI can handle the activities of daily living to a limited degree if they pace themselves. Athletes are trained to pace themselves. The same should be true for those who perform ordinary everyday activities. Pacing your work over several hours may get you through the tasks of the day without incurring increasing pain that forces you to stop work entirely.

Share Your Chores

Many of my RSI patients can be helped to maintain their households by sharing chores when they find they can no longer do them alone. Divide chores by abilities, so that you get to do the ones that don't cause you pain or difficulty. Another answer may be to delegate chores when possible. It is infuriating for an injured person who is in pain to have his or her children or spouse refuse to help out. A delicate balance needs to be struck between having to share your chores with members of your family and having them become caretakers. A serious discussion about the role of the household members needs to take place. This kind of family interaction can be an emotional struggle, and professional help may be needed.

If You Live Alone

Be inventive in doing your household chores. Perhaps setting slightly lower standards of neatness by letting go for a while and pacing yourself would be a desirable means of coping. For women, modify your hairstyle to a wash-and-wear style. Give up panty hose–they're too hard to pull on and off. Wear slip-on shoes with wedge-shaped, nearly flat heels and Velcro closures. Men should consider growing a well-kept beard if they can't shave easily. When you get new clothing, opt for items that you can put on easily, such as with elastic waists and loosely fit.

If You Can, Hire a Housekeeper, Cook, or Helper

When you are ill or disabled, a helper ceases to be a luxury. A great burden of work can be lifted if there is someone to clean, cook, or do chores–and there are resources for people who can't afford to hire someone on their own. Meals that can be prescribed by your physician from social agencies or your church group and part-time helpers from organizations such as the Visiting Nurses Association may be means of coping. RSI self-help groups may be able to identify other resources. Refer to the Internet resources section for more information.

The Telephone

If you are using the phone a lot, a headset should always be attached to the phone. Patients report that this is especially important in the kitchen, where the hands are occupied with cooking chores. Headsets also come in a cordless form. Various types of headphones are available from the Hello Direct Catalog (1-800-444-3556) or from Staples and Radio Shack, among others.

Cellular phones are becoming commonplace replacements for the home phone. Gripping these tiny phones while holding them to your ear and tilting your head is similar to holding a computer mouse to your ear–uncomfortable for anyone, not just RSI sufferers. Earpieces can ease the muscular burden.

Voice dialing is available from most phone companies. Technological advances in phoning are occurring rapidly, and phones now have caller ID and number storage that dial with the press of a single button. Keep yourself informed about other work-saving services available from your phone company

Sleeping

Sleep promotes healing. Normally, we all spend a third of our lives in bed. Unfortunately, the time you spend reading in bed can only contribute to your problems if you are injuring yourself while you do it. Most people with RSI have postural problems involving their necks. Curving your spine and neck to see the TV screen or reading a book when your hands hurt and you can't support the book doubles your trouble. Learn to sit while you read or watch television. Save your bed for restorative sleep, sexual activity, and relaxation.

Positioning yourself for restorative sleep involves protecting your arms, keeping them relaxed, and not bending at the elbow or wrist. Some people can do this by sleeping on their backs with pillow supports under each arm. An easier method is to use soft cushioning as a splint (only while you sleep) to limit the bending of elbows and wrists. This can be achieved by wrapping your arms in cotton rolls under a loose elastic bandage. Your health care provider can help you find the right solution.

The words "restorative sleep" are to be taken seriously; get as close to eight hours a night as you can, but don't spend all your time in bed. When depressed, people often spend a lot of time in bed, but their sleep is fitful and not restorative. If you feel your sleep disturbance is due to depression, you should consult a psychiatrist. If you are seeing more than one physician, be sure each knows what medications you are taking.

Sleeping medications have both positive and negative effects on people with RSI. While they can help you get to sleep, almost all aids for sleeping disturb REM sleep, which is necessary for restorative sleep. If you use sleep medications, but find you are nevertheless restless and waking up during the night, try to cut down on the pills with your physician's supervision, as withdrawal symptoms are possible. Caffeine and alcoholic beverages also can disturb healthful sleep and should be limited.

Sexual Activity

Sex may pose a problem if you have RSI, and here you have to turn to both practical and inventive solutions. We all need love and affection, and sexual activity is naturally a part of our emotional lives. Fortunately, we live in a time where we can find solutions in the library or advice from professional sources. As in other aspects of RSI, there are solutions to the physical limitations you are experiencing. Keep in mind that affectionate conversation with your partner will do more to help your sex life than acrimonious confrontation.

Relaxation

The very fact that you have RSI may indicate that you are normally a busy, active, or tense person. Learning to let go and relax is one of your tasks. High stress levels can affect your recovery and your therapy. Some activities that have helped our patients relax include music, theater, dance, self-awareness programs, body awareness programs, meditation, modified yoga, retreats or vacations, and lifestyle changes that can mean anything from modifying the way you work, to changing your job, to moving to a new location, to changing your exercise and diet regimen. Seek the help of a mental health professional to guide you to activities that will relax you. See chapter 3 for more information.

Reading

In my experience, the last activity to improve during recovery is the ability to read comfortably holding a book or newspaper. A reading stand or a special pillow to prop up the book is available from sources such as the Levenger Company (1-800-544-0880). You simply can't turn pages? Books on tape are useful for RSI sufferers. Slip-on rubber fingers also are useful for turning pages. Special book weights can be used to hold books open for reading.

Hand and Finger Movement

Most of my patients who developed RSI doing computer work also have difficulty with handwriting. Here are a few pointers that can help. Certain pens are easier to use than others. A standard ballpoint requires uncomfortably tight gripping and pressing. Fat pens are available for better gripping. A fountain pen with a smooth-flowing point can be easier to use than a typical ballpoint pen. Vera Wills recommends the Pilot Precise V7 fine rolling ball pen because it flows easily across the paper, and there are other brands of "rolling ball" pens as well. A sponge hair curler also can help ease the strain of gripping the pen (see figure 25). As with any other activity, writing requires that you pace yourself. Use printed address labels so you don't have to keep writing your return address on bills and documents. If you write to someone regularly, make your own mailing labels. Voice-activated computer technology may be useful for home computer work and help with bill paying as well as writing. See the details in chapter 8. An electric stapler, electric scissors, and an electric letter opener will help save your hands. Use self-adhesive stamps and envelopes to minimize the chore of pressing.

In the Kitchen

A phone with a headset or a hands-free speakerphone is essential kitchen communication equipment. Paper plates and plastic utensils can be bought in bulk and used to avoid washing dishes. If you insist on washing dishes, get a dishwashing sponge with a soap-filled handle. Soak the dishes before you clean them. An automatic dishwasher can also be helpful, but of course it requires loading and unloading.

Use the type of Chinese cutting knife that has two handles, allowing you to rock it through the food you are cutting. Buy an electric can opener and a light iron, and look into various types of ergonomic kitchen utensils, including those that are designed for arthritics. The Oxo Company makes tools with soft handles that are available in household stores. Special jar openers also are available. Remember to dip the jar caps in hot water before opening. Scissors used in the kitchen should have spring-loaded handles. When buying groceries, buy small sizes if you have to carry them, or get an easy-to-push four-wheeled shopping cart. If possible, have your groceries delivered. If you redesign your kitchen, seek the help of a disability specialist or ergonomist who might recommend changing counter heights, setting up foot pedal faucets, or changing doorknobs to the easier-to-open lever type.

In the Bathroom

Electric toothbrushes are available that can be held with a fist grip if your thumb hurts. Lightweight hair dryers also are available. Taking a shower instead of a bath can avoid the strain of getting into and pulling yourself out of your tub. Look into changing the water taps to the lever kind they use in hospitals and installing handle grips to help you get in and out of the shower or tub. Use wall dispensers for shampoo and other liquids.

Driving

For most of us, the car is indispensable, but for a person with RSI, driving can become difficult or impossible. Cars are not the ergonomic triumphs that many manufacturers would have us believe. We may sit slumped in the car seat, often forced to look up or down depending on our body build and how much headroom the car allows us. Since RSI is essentially an upper-body illness, the various activities of driving—moving the neck in various directions. gripping the wheel and moving it, shifting gears, and getting in and out of the vehicle—all can trigger symptoms or even cause a relapse during recovery. Be practical in your choice of vehicle. Driving an SUV means you are adding to your physical burden by pulling yourself up into the vehicle and driving a small truck. Try items that have worked for others, such as foam cushioning on the steering wheel, wheelchair gloves, or lumbar support pillows to keep you propped up at the steering wheel. Electronically adjustable seats should be something to look for if you are getting a new car.

Become a passenger whenever you can. If you go on long trips and are driving, stop by the roadside every forty-five minutes to an hour to rest for five to ten minutes. Know your limitations—don't wait for pain to tell you to stop. If you can only drive for thirty minutes before the onset of symptoms, stop after twenty minutes. Resume driving only after a sufficient rest break, which you can determine by experience.

You will have to add your own tips to the ones in this chapter. Be inventive about the things you absolutely must do, and give up the things you can dispense with. Above all, take help where you can get it, and remember to save your upper body for home exercises and the important work of getting better.

11

Getting Back to Work

It is the Age of Machinery, in every outward and inward sense of that word.

—Thomas Carlyle (1795–1881), *Signs of the Times*

The field of occupational medicine had its beginning in the eighteenth century, when Bernardino Ramazzini studied people at work and used that knowledge to describe a type of physical illness that had never been reported before his time. As result of his work published in 1713, he is considered the father of occupational medicine. Were Ramazzini around today, he would note that the computer's flat keyboard has created a work hazard far greater than what occurred with the invention of the typewriter.

In 1808, Pellegrino Turri made, for a blind friend, what is probably the first mechanical typewriter. Commercial production began in 1870 with the invention of the writing ball by a Danish poet and part-time inventor named Malling Hansen. The modern mechanical typewriter dates to 1873, when Sholes and Glidden introduced the first typewriter with a QWERTY keyboard, manufactured for the American market by the Remington Arms Company.

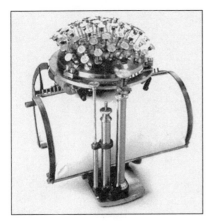

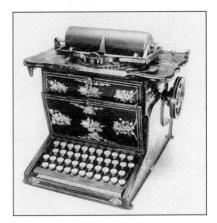

Figure 38. The Malling Hansen writing ball

Figure 39. The Sholes and Glidden typewriter, the world's first commercially successful typewriter

The QWERTY keyboard was designed to separate frequently used type bars so that they could not lock together when struck. While the stepped keyboard of the mechanical typewriter is gone, we still have the QWERTY layout, now on a flattened electronic keyboard, which became popular in the early 1980s with the introduction of the PC. Attempts to introduce other keyboard configurations such as the DVORAK layout (see figure 40) have not been generally accepted, although those who have learned the DVORAK claim it is far more comfortable than the standard configuration. Whacking away at a standard typewriter's stepped mechanical keyboard did not cre-

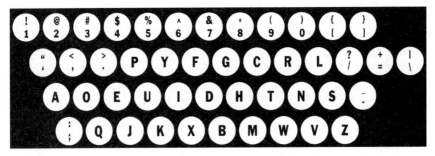

Figure 40. The Dvorak keyboard, an idea that didn't quite catch on

ate the injuries we see today, because the typist had to use more of the upper body than we now use tapping the flat keys with only our forearms and hands. Excessive work at the mechanical typewriter was more likely to produce sore shoulders.

Frederick Winslow Taylor was a highly educated engineer who developed a number of industrial innovations, including time-and-motion study. His book *Principles of Scientific Management,* published in the late nineteenth century, led to the high-speed assembly line, stripping work of many of its rewarding aspects. His concepts were adopted worldwide, and established him as the father of scientific management. Work became harder, more boring, faster, and more stressful for industrial workers and office workers, yet his work is one of the basic approaches to industry today. He was the first real efficiency expert.

The concept of Taylorism, and the flat computer keyboard, which can respond faster than any typist can key, exposed office workers to the illnesses of repetitive motion as never before. This was further aggravated by the introduction of the mouse and the CRT monitor, which added to the dimensions of injury.

The personal computer has now been an integral part of our daily lives for at least the past twenty years, and to deal with the workplace injuries resulting from its use, the Occupational Safety and Health Administration (OSHA) issued standards and rules to protect employees from RSI in many industries. Employers in general considered these rules too costly, despite California's successful adoption of a similar set of rules. In January 2001, the National Academy of Sciences, issued a report called "Musculoskeletal Disorders and the Workplace," which stated that 1 million injuries were caused by repetitive motions on the job along with other work-related ergonomic factors. The report stated that a conservative estimate of the cost of these injuries was $50 billion a year. According to an article in the *New York Times,* "some corporate groups estimated that the new rules would cost $120 billion while OSHA put the cost at $4.5 billion."

When employers realize that they can save money by preventing RSI, we should then see more adoption of prevention programs. There are enlightened employers known in the health care community for their pioneering approach to prevention—L. L. Bean, Blue Cross/Blue Shield of California, the *New York Times,* and the *Los Angeles Times,* among many others.

If an injury reporting system is set up to flag ergonomic trouble spots, the potential problems can be identified and corrected. There are many highly successful employee injury prevention programs that have produced a marked decrease in employee injury, and studies have shown that industry predictions about the costs of a preventive program are often far off target. Companies that employ full- or part-time physical therapists and that provide fitness facilities have fewer RSI problems among their staff. Small businesses can enlist community facilities as a support system for prevention programs and can contract for ergonomic consultation services.

The workers' compensation system, which may differ slightly from state to state, is an insurance program established, in part, to pay for the medical care of injured workers. If you are filing for workers' compensation benefits call your local office, ask questions, and obtain informational literature from them. Unions, some companies, and local RSI self-help groups distribute workers' compensation information. Remember that the trade-off when receiving workers' compensation benefits is that when you sign on to the system, your right to sue your employer is markedly diminished.

Recent studies suggest that many people are reluctant to report RSI to the workers' compensation system. One article reports that only one in every eleven injuries is actually reported. In my own experience, 60 percent of RSI patients continued to work despite the fact that they were injured.

Unfortunately, the workers' compensation system has many flaws. Physicians are generally paid low fees, which is a disincentive to perform the thorough examination necessary for the proper diagnosis of RSI. Workers' comp physicians are often surgical specialists who are faced with treating RSI, a nonsurgical illness. Often, workers' comp physicians balk at attributing the patient's injury to work—all too often the case when independent medical examiners (IMEs) are required to substantiate a diagnosis. IMEs are employed by insurance companies to protect the insurance companies from fraud and simply to save money, which can create a conflict of interest. For a variety of reasons, the patient is often thwarted in his or her attempt to prove the relationship of his or her injury to work. Bureaucratic entanglement causes delays, and patients can wait months before being certified for treatment.

If your workers' compensation claim is not approved, it's time to think about an attorney. In a contested case, the insurance company will have a representative at your hearing. It is wise to have someone representing you. The attorney you choose should be experienced in workers' compensation litigation.

Back to Work

Once you have RSI and are in treatment, you will have to start thinking about returning to full- or part-time work, the most difficult nonhealth-related challenge you will face with RSI. To achieve a return to normal function, there are certain goals that you will need to meet.

You must participate actively in your rehabilitation. Passive participation simply will not be enough to get you through your treatment. No therapist can do your home therapy for you, and you make no progress without your home or gym work. Maintaining the stretching and strengthening exercises is what advances your professionally supervised therapy.

You will have to learn by trial and error to limit both work and nonwork activities before you feel pain. One way to do this is to time an activity and note when you begin to feel uncomfortable or feel pain. Limit this activity to a few minutes short of the onset of pain the next time you do the activity, and become aware of the feeling you get when pain is about to ensue. With activities of daily living, you have to discipline yourself so you don't schedule more than you can achieve. Above all, you must attain and maintain good posture, because we know that bad posture is a trigger for harmful injuries of RSI.

An important part of retraining is to note what your upper body feels like when it is no longer tight, and when the larger muscles of your upper back begin to work in conjunction with the shoulder, arm, and hand muscles. This sense memory should be recalled whenever you are exercising. You must limit pressure on neck and shoulder muscles and nerves, which means you should no longer carry heavy knapsacks, shoulder bags, briefcases, or shopping bags.

You must become aware of awkward positioning and activities during retraining. Even seemingly minor things such as keeping your nails short is important so you avoid inefficient use of your hands. Take sufficient rest breaks from any potentially harmful activities. Five to ten minutes every hour for office workers is a good idea.

Retraining for work should be done in a structured and orderly fashion so there is a gradual resumption of activities that previously caused symptoms. Know your limits: getting an idea of the severity of your injury is very important and can be useful in helping you determine whether you are ready to return to work. Impulsive behavior and a rapid return to full activity because you are feeling better can lead to a flare-up and delay recovery.

Adherence to your rehabilitation program and your awareness of the extent of your injury will keep you from a major relapse. Rehabilitation will probably take longer than you like, and you may have an occasional relapse, but keep at it!

People you work with may become problems. If they don't understand what you are going through, they may resent having to pick up some of the slack from you. If you are recovering from RSI and have returned to work, you may feel pressure to resume your usual pace. Don't do it. Instead, try to make your fellow workers understand what you are going through.

The Case of Dr. M

Dr. M is a devoted and conscientious eye surgeon who specializes in cataract operations. For several weeks each year, he spent time in developing countries removing cataracts from those otherwise unable to afford the operation. Cataract surgery involves intensive and delicate use of the hands and fingers, and absolute control is required to release the clouded lens and to suture the wound with tiny stitches. Dr. M does this work almost continuously all day long, crouching over the patient through most of the work. Over time, this took its toll on his posture, leading to the cascade of events common in RSI patients.

When he came to me, he was in constant pain and visibly upset because he could no longer work effectively. He saw his career "going down the tubes." He had been to see his primary care physician, who referred him to an orthopedic surgeon. Dr. M followed the suggestions of the orthopedist, but his condition did not improve. In fact, even though he wasn't working, his symptoms got worse. Other physicians he consulted told him he had RSI and suggested rest and nonsteroidal anti-inflammatory medications. These had only marginal effects.

When I first saw him, he was somewhat skeptical of the ability of his fellow physicians to help, and he considered me his last resort. I spent a great deal of time on his examination, explaining what I was doing all along the way. The evaluation showed typical findings. Over the years, his posture had deteriorated, his head was thrust forward, and the compression and traction of the nerves in his neck had caused pain in his arm and hands. I offered him specific diagnoses and recommended he work with a physical therapist whose specialty was RSI. At the end of the exam I sensed that he was still dubious. Nevertheless, he began working with the therapist, who did soft-tissue work and started Dr. M on a series of focused home exercises and strengthening activities.

After about a month, Dr. M. reported improvement. After six months, he was able to resume a full work schedule while continuing his exercise and strengthening program. Dr. M also made some changes in the way he set himself up at the operating table. He got into a more comfortable and ergonomically less harmful position. He paced himself and made other lifestyle changes. The letter of thanks I received from him was touching, and I had the satisfaction of knowing I had helped bring back a physician who was now able to continue his important work.

Are You Ready to Return?

Here are some criteria you can use to determine your level of symptoms and capabilities in judging whether you can return to work or other activities. These are helpful but are only to be used as a rough guide.

Completely Limited

Here you are unable to perform any activities of daily living or work activities without setting off symptoms that may last weeks or even months. These symptoms are usually constant and include aches, pain, numbness, tingling, and spasms. Obviously, return to work is out of the question.

Very Limited

You can awake pain-free and perform four or five arm-related activities before the onset of pain and other symptoms. These symptoms can last for several hours, decrease with rest, and increase with further hand activity. The symptoms are usually gone by the next day. Return to work cannot proceed easily under these circumstances.

Moderately Limited

For brief periods, you can perform activities of daily living and work-related activities without the onset of symptoms. You are free of pain most of the time except after strenuous hand and arm activity. A low level of sustained activity is tolerated, but if limits are exceeded, pain may last for the next day or two. If this is your situation, limited work with numerous rest breaks is possible provided discipline is maintained.

Mildly Limited

You are pain-free most of the time unless activities are pushed beyond ordinary functional levels. Accordingly, short deadlines and binge work must be avoided. Work is possible, but only after establishing the need for these limitations with the employer and fellow employees who may feel they are carrying your load.

The Difficult Activities

If you are in constant pain and having difficulty deciding which activities are likely to cause you the most trouble during your rehabilitation, this list of particularly harmful activities compiled by our patients can be useful:

- Carrying a heavy backpack
- Putting on makeup
- Combing or blowdrying hair
- Sexual activity
- Cooking
- Shaking hands
- Holding a book or newspaper
- Shopping, carrying groceries
- Knitting
- Using a scissors
- Opening mail
- Vacuuming
- Pulling a shopping cart
- Walking the dog
- Pulling doorknobs
- Washing dishes
- Putting on clothing
- Writing

Computer Problems

Certain kinds of computer use are more challenging than others, and more likely to cause pain.

- Artists who do computer graphics and who probably are at greater risk for injury because of intensive mouse use

- Architects and draftsmen who use special input devices such as the "puck," which has numerous buttons

- Typists who do data input work, particularly if they are subject to deadlines and binge work

- Telephone operators who transcribe telephone calls for the deaf

- Typists who do television subtitles for the deaf, or who provide directory information

- Temporary word processors who work under time pressure and who must go from one temporary workstation to another

- Anyone who must keep a fast and constant pace

The Functional Capacity Evaluation

Occasionally, during your illness or just about when you are ready to return to work, you may be asked by your insurance provider to submit to a functional capacity evaluation, a standardized test that purports to establish your ability to return to work. In many instances this testing is done too soon or does not evaluate some of the actual things you will be doing. Obviously, if this test is performed on a severely injured person, it is a foregone conclusion that the result of the test will not be helpful except to establish a baseline. Often the testing itself can provoke a relapse. A functional capacity evaluation, usually done by an occupational therapist, is designed to describe the individual's current lifestyle and observe his or her performance with appropriate levels of work-related tasks. These include tests of arm dexterity, upper-extremity coordination, and the effect of speed on function. The examination also tests strength in gripping, pinching, lifting, and carrying, and makes observations of mobility, static posture, weight-bearing ability, and balance.

From these observations, conclusions are drawn about your ability to return to work and what the limitations of that work might be. These tests are abstracts of standard capabilities and may not reflect what you actually do at work.

Returning to work is not a decision to be taken lightly. Although most people are eager to get back, returning too early can be disastrous. It is worth the effort to give careful consideration to your physical state before you decide to go back.

12

RSI and Musicians

Music, the greatest good that mortals know, and all of heaven we have below.

–Joseph Addison (1672–1719), "A Song for St. Cecilia's Day"

My interest in RSI began in a facility I established for the treatment of injured musicians. Musicians need physical conditioning, but this fact is often ignored in the traditional music schools and conservatories. Music pedagogy is very traditional and still relies on the many years of experience passed down through generations. We are losing many talented musicians to injury early in their careers because they (and their teachers) ignore the need for physical conditioning and lack the necessary knowledge to use biomechanically correct technique to prevent injury. Dancers, on the other hand, have learned that just dancing is not enough to keep them in shape and prevent injury. This is why we see dancers doing weight training, stretching, and strengthening exercises. Those lucky musical students who are in an enlightened training environment are doing these exercises, too.

By applying concepts of physical conditioning, ergonomics, and biomechanics, musicians can not only prevent injury but also gain a competitive edge: the quality of the music delivered will improve because of better positioning, greater strength, and finer muscular control.

When a physical examination is performed on an injured musician we are likely to find the same kinds of problems that we have described in this book for computer users and other workers, with only slight differences. Emotionally speaking, musicians are very caught up in their music; when an injury occurs it can be psychologically devastating, threatening to undo years of study and hard work. The ergonomic and biomechanical aspects of the treatment of musicians are very specific. Biomechanical retraining, something akin to technique training, is better managed with the help of a knowledgeable fellow musician who can communicate more easily with the injured musician, especially when it comes to changes in fingering or repertoire. With a combination of musical biomechanical retraining and the physical and occupational therapy that is always required in RSI injury, the results can be spectacular.

Which Musicians Get Injured?

If we look at the group of musicians who came to our facility in the first two years of its operation, we can see that piano and string instrument injuries predominate. This suggests that these very popular instruments pose the greatest ergonomic and biomechanical challenges. Of course, it is also possible that there are simply more people playing these particular instruments than others.

Here is a breakdown of 401 musicians in a study I performed who sustained injury as a result of playing their instrument over a two-year period:

Instrument	No. of Musicians Injured per Instrument
Keyboard	
piano	133
harpsichord	3
organ	1
Total	137 (34 percent of musician injuries)
Woodwind/Brass	
flute	13
oboe	6
clarinet	9
saxophone	2
bassoon	4
French horn	9
trumpet	4
trombone	3
Total	50 (12 percent of musician injuries)
Percussion	
drums	29
vibraphone	1
Total	30 (7 percent of musician injuries)
Strings	
violin	81
guitar	66
viola	16
double bass	13
harp	5
Total	181 (45 percent of musician injuries)

(continued)

Instrument	No. of Musicians Injured per Instrument
Others	
accordion	1
conductor	2
Total	3 (0.7 percent of musician injuries)

The Ergonomics of Musical Instruments

In Greek mythology, Procrustes invited his guests to sleep in his bed, which he claimed was exactly the right size for each of them. What he didn't tell them was the way in which he made the bed fit: by stretching his guests on a rack if they were too short, or cutting off their legs if they were too tall. Like Procrustes' guests, many musicians find themselves trying to adapt to an instrument, instead of adapting the instrument to themselves.

Some instruments, such as the piano or string instruments, don't lend themselves easily to substantial physical modifications. Yet breakthroughs can occur. On November 4, 1997, an article appeared in the *Wall Street Journal* about a young woman's quest for a narrower keyboard. Hannah Riemann, a five-foot-tall, ninety-eight-pound piano teacher and pianist with small hands, wrote to many companies attempting to persuade them to make a piano with narrower keys so she could play more comfortably. Almost all companies refused, citing high production costs for little profit. Some even considered this an "inconsequential, ridiculous thought" or "an imaginary problem." When she was a youngster, her teachers assured her she would grow into the standard keyboard, but she never did. Apparently her problem is not unique. Yoshimo Nakada, one of Japan's most popular composers, and the Viennese pianist,

Paul Badura, have voiced similar concerns. At one point, Ms. Riemann learned that Kawai and Yamaha, Japanese piano manufacturers, listed narrow keyboard pianos in their catalogs, but that they were only available on a limited basis in Japan. Finally, she persuaded the German company that makes keyboard parts for Steinway to make her a narrow prototype that slides into a standard piano and lines up to strike the strings properly. Her keyboard is about four inches shorter than the standard length. (In the nineteenth century, octave width was $1/4$ inch narrower than it is today because the keys were $15/16$ inch narrower.) With her new setup, Ms. Riemann can play "anything, even Rachmaninoff," with greater ease.

Other, less dramatic attempts at ergonomic improvement of musical instruments include Vladimir Horowitz's insistence on traveling with his own Steinway, probably so he could have consistent keyboard touch. Other performers travel with their own benches. But these are ergonomic luxuries usually denied to ordinary musicians.

Violists are another group of musicians who have benefited from ergonomic changes in their instruments. The viola is a larger version of the violin, and an ergonomically deficient cause of injury. Here the credit goes to David Lloyd Rivinus for creating the Pellegrina Viola and the Maximilian Violin. He has lightened the instrument, adjusted string angle, made the instrument asymmetrical for comfort, provided setup adjustments to accommodate different-size hands, changed tailpiece design, and added extra sound holes. So far he has made twenty-seven violas, and is increasing production on the violins. Mr. Rivinus can be reached at riviola@blueskyweb.com or at 503-925-1628 (phone) or 503-925-0410 (fax).

The double bass, the viola, the violin, the cello, and other instruments can vary in size, so that choosing the right instrument is extremely important. Flutes, clarinets, oboes, bassoons, French horns, and many other instruments can have their keys modified to make them more comfortable. You don't wear one-size-fits-all shoes; a musician shouldn't have to play a one-size-fits-all instrument.

Beyond some modest changes in the form of the instrument, the only practical way to avoid injury is to do what we are proposing for the nonmusicians in this book. There is a myth among musicians that exercising may actually be harmful, making the musician "muscle-bound" and causing a loss of dexterity. Nothing could be farther from the truth. The musician must regard himself as an athlete, maintain proper posture and strength, and use a proper ergonomic and biomechanical approach. The less ergonomically adaptable the instrument, the more the instrumentalist will have to pay attention to the biomechanical aspects of playing. Following is a brief discussion of the various musical instruments, the problems they present, and some suggestions to help overcome their difficulties.

Piano, Harpsichord, Organ

In this group of instruments, physical conditioning and posture need particular attention by the musician. Correct posture and distance from the keyboard as well as light touch and properly curved fingers are helpful in reducing soft-tissue trauma. While doing her Ed.D. thesis, my associate Yu-Pin Hsu, an occupational therapist and musician, studied fifty pianists and found that postural misalignment was present in more than 90 percent and thoracic outlet syndrome in 80 percent. Poor technique was consistently observed.

Computer keys, electronic keys, and organ keys bottom out to a hard surface with minimal cushioning, but piano keys don't. Hitting uncushioned keys too hard is the equivalent of a ballet dancer working on a concrete surface, instead of a sprung or cushioned floor, which is now standard for dance stages (and wrestling rings!). The organist has the additional problem of playing on several keyboards and the need to work pedal bars as well. This requires strength and coordination in the lower body as it works with the upper extremities. The organ seat is often not adjustable.

Fifty Injured Pianists: A Research Project

In 1997, my assistant Yu-Pin Hsu devoted her Ed. D. thesis to an analysis of factors contributing to the development of RSI in pianists. First, she used examination data we had recorded on 50 pianists ranging in age from 18 to 64 years, 29 of whom were males. The subjects consisted of 22 professional pianists, 8 teachers, 14 students, and 6 recreational pianists. Their common symptom was pain related to their piano playing. Forty-seven pianists were right-handed. Twenty-eight exercised regularly, 13 occasionally, and 9 never. In addition to pain, 9 reported weakness and fatigue, 6 had tingling in the hands, 5 had numbness, and 4 had tightness and stiffness in the arms and hands. One person lost finger coordination, and 1 had tremors. They practiced an average of 3.6 hours a day, with a range from a few minutes to 8 hours a day.

Dr. Hsu set about videotaping all of these musicians as they played a standard repertoire. Aberrant postures, awkward positioning, and other potentially harmful technique idiosyncrasies were recorded. These are the results of her observations:

Fingers: Hyperextension of the pianists' fingers was demonstrated in 46 of 50 subjects. Hyperextension is known to be an inefficient way to use the fingers (see chapter 9).

Wrists: Awkward positioning of the wrists contributes to injury by overworking the forearm muscles. Forty-seven people showed excessive wrist ulnar deviation. Ten showed radial deviation. Eight either flexed or extended their wrists excessively. Twenty-six showed wrist motion unnecessary to carrying out their musical repertoire.

Forearms: Elbows held too close to the body caused two main problems: forcing the pianist to compensate by going into ulnar deviation, and limiting range of motion. Twenty subjects held their elbows too close to the body. Two people held their forearms in excessive supination, and 2 played in hyperpronation.

Other upper extremity activities: In addition to playing

the piano, other upper extremity activities were affected negatively, including a tendency to drop objects.

Diagnostic data: Postural misalignment and RSI were found to be the main problems in 49 subjects. Forty-three had protracted shoulders. Head and neck problems, scapular winging, and other upper and lower back problems also were common.

Harp

There is little one can do ergonomically with a standard harp except to use a smaller or a larger version. In my experience, the main problem for harpists is poor physical conditioning combined with lack of shoulder and upper arm involvement in plucking strings. Excessive wrist motion in ulnar and radial deviation and poor position, particularly as the hand is placed in dorsiflexion, lead to forearm muscle overuse, particularly when combined with the common postural problems seen in RSI.

Violin

Biomechanically this instrument is a challenge, but certain adjustments can make playing the violin a lot more comfortable. It is important to be sure that the chin rests and shoulder rests are suitable to the length of the player's neck. A long neck will require the shoulder rest to be set high. There are many different types of shoulder rests, but nearly all of them do not fill what I call the "forgotten space" just under the clavicle or collarbone. When this "forgotten space" is not filled, the violin will angle forward and tend to fall off the shoulder. The musician compensates by gripping the neck of the violin tightly with the left thumb and pressing down with his neck. This tightening of the thumb also makes it harder to flex and extend the rest of the fingers and can lead to injury. An easy solution is to place a soft sponge in the form of a wedge, which fills the "forgotten space" and stabilizes the instrument. This should set the body of the violin at about a thirty-degree downward angle from the horizontal. This enables the bow to work the strings steadily and more horizontally. With the help of gravity, bowing is smoother, and to that extent the quality of the music is improved. The chin rest may be more comfortable if centrally placed over the tailpiece of the violin, so that the musician faces forward. Relieving the pressure on the neck will additionally prevent the common chronic inflammation of the skin know as "fiddler's neck."

Viola

The viola is essentially a bigger violin and can cause problems because of its size. The viola should be chosen with consideration of both the player's size and the sound quality of the instrument. Good instruments 16 or 16½ inches in length are available, while the larger 17-inch instrument, which might be chosen for its sound, has greater potential for injury. A sponge wedge under the "forgotten space" below the clavicle is as useful for the viola as it is for the violin. An ergonomic viola has been created that reshapes the body of the viola in an asymmetrical form, placing more of it away from the neck to allow more freedom of movement. (See figure 41.)

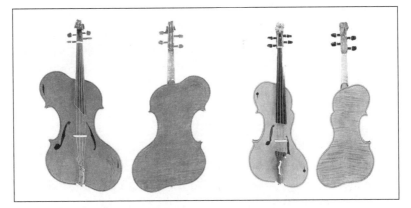

Figure 41. The modified Pellegrina viola (left) and the Maximilian violin

Cello

Proper positioning of the cello certainly demands good physical conditioning in the upper body and specifically in the entire back. Low back problems are common among cellists, often because proper seating is not given enough attention. Positioning may also be modified by the use of a bent floor pin, such as the one designed by master cellist and conductor Mstislav Rostropovich. The flatter configuration of the instrument, sometimes with the use of a bent pin, allows the bow to be assisted by gravity, improving the quality of the music as well as enhancing comfort. If the pegs tuning the string tension get in the way of the left side of your head, they can be eliminated by substituting a keyhole and removable key arrangement similar to that of a clock's winding mechanism. Cello width also should be taken into consideration when choosing an instrument. An occupational illness known as cellist's scrotum has been described as the result of the instrument rubbing the crotch of the musician.

Double Bass

This is an instrument whose huge size poses ergonomic problems even in transporting it. Rather than using a shoulder strap, many musicians push it around on a large wheel attached to the case. The instrument sits on a pin and is played by either plucking or bowing the strings. An instrument this large requires the musician to be in optimal physical condition to avoid injury. Larger body size is helpful, but not entirely necessary. There are various size instruments that can be fitted for comfort for people of different sizes and shapes. The most common problems I've encountered with double bass players are postural misalignment, neurogenic thoracic outlet syndrome, and low back syndrome.

Guitar

Classical guitars are light but unwieldy and are somewhat difficult to stabilize. A good, wide shoulder strap can help. Guitars may be held in a variety of positions while sitting or standing, which further complicates playing the instrument. When sitting, the classical position, with the body of the instrument centrally located and the left leg elevated, is ergonomically efficient, since it allows both wrists to be held in a neutral position. This is what we suggest when treating injured players, even those using heavy rock bass guitars. In the sitting position, various devices from sponges to rubber mats are used to stabilize the body of the instrument on the left knee (for a right-handed player). An A-frame holder for the thighs also is available. Finally, lighter strings, in the 9- to 10-gauge range, offer less tension and are useful in the early stage of retraining an injured player. Electric guitars and bass instruments have problems relating to both weight and positioning. In the standing position, the instrument should be centered and held low enough so that both the right and the left wrist can achieve neutral positioning.

Percussion

The percussion instruments usually involve vigorous physical activity that you might think would keep the musician in good physical shape. And in fact, we see percussionists less often than most. Nevertheless they can get hurt if their biomechanical technique is poor. The most common flaw in drummers was presented by A. P., a self-taught rock drummer who was able to pursue his career without any problems until he hit his midthirties. As aging affected his posture, he began to notice diminished strength in his arms coupled with pain during and after a concert. When I first examined him I noticed, apart from his round-shouldered posture, that he was gripping his drumsticks very tightly, locking his shoulders in place, and essentially using only wrist motion to perform. Even though he looked quite strong, he was essentially losing the considerable strength and movement available in his upper arms and shoulders. I have seen this not only in drummers but also in injured tympanists, xylophonists, and vibraphone players, among others. An analogy for this wrist-only technique would be a baseball pitcher trying to throw a fastball by flicking his wrist. When A. P. saw the videotape we made of him at the drums, he was shocked. He never realized how badly he was limiting his upper body movement. We began his retraining by having him repeat the motion of drumming while integrating shoulder movement into his stroke. Joe Morello, a master drummer and teacher formerly with Dave Brubeck's group, gave me this tip: use your upper body the same way you would if you were slapping your thighs. We built on this concept, and soon after stretching and strengthening exercises, postural retraining, and some ergonomic guidance, A. P.'s strength increased enormously, and shortly thereafter, an almost magical transformation took place. A. P. is again regularly performing dynamic drum solos for his rock group—and without pain.

Flute

This instrument can be extremely injurious. Luckily, the flute, along with several other wind instruments, is eminently amenable to substantial changes to make it more comfortable to play. Most of the factory-produced instruments simply do not fit most hands. Some work I did with a flutist is a good example of the ways in which an instrument can be modified.

A young woman came to see me because, while she had been playing the flute for ten years, it was nevertheless very uncomfortable, even painful, for her to continue to play it. After a complete examination it was obvious that while she was in good general health, she did have congenital shortening of the fourth and fifth fingers of both hands. I placed her in a biomechanically correct position, and took measurements between the keys she could not reach and her fingers. I carefully placed the flute on a copying machine and drew the new key configuration with Wite-Out. I then took the instrument to a technician, who soft-soldered new extensions as in the diagram. When the patient returned, she was fitted with a temporary support based on the web space between the thumb and index finger until she got used to her new position (see figure 42). A "crutch" to widen her grip was placed on the body of the instrument. With minor adjustments to increase comfort, she was eventually able to play comfortably.

Another technique recently used (with the help of Vera Wills, a musical ergonomist) was to attach adhesive-backed felt on the keys for the musician to try while undergoing retraining. In this case, a flutist who had quit the stage was able to return to performing after these modifications were made permanent.

Problems with the flute relate particularly to the left hand, where the wrist is forced upward into dorsiflexion and radial deviation, while the index finger is further extended at the knuckle and then is severely flexed at the second joint. In addition, the third, fourth, and fifth fingers often have to be stretched or extended to reach the keys. The stress put on muscles and

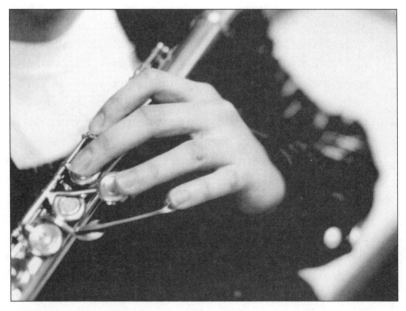

Figure 42. A modified flute

tendons by these positions is enormous and can lead to severe problems, especially in people with small hands or short fingers. Modifications like the ones we describe here put the wrist in a neutral position and allow the other fingers to be comfortably curved, offering a relaxed posture and better control. Other devices, such as support stands for the whole instrument or a curved-neck flute, can be useful in overcoming some of the ergonomic problems faced by the flutist. The approach to modifying use of the piccolo is similar but less often required.

Keeping the flutist facing forward while playing is worth the retraining effort to diminish neck twisting and bending for both increased comfort and related postural problems.

Occasionally flutists will develop focal dystonia in their fingers or embouchure muscles. Focal dystonia, also known as writer's cramp, is one of the worst occupational injuries a musician can face. When it occurs, years of study and a livelihood can be put in peril or completely extinguished. Usually there is severe emotional upset associated with this catastrophic event. There are many ways in which musicians affected with focal dystonia cope with their illness. A flutist with dystonia of the muscles surrounding the mouth (the orbicularis oris) might be able to switch to an instrument with a different embouchure, such as a clarinet. This ability to function with a different instrument tells us that focal dystonia is task-specific. A violinist with focal dystonia might attempt to change the position of the instrument and undergo biomechanical retraining to attempt to regain control of his or her fingers. In my experience this is possible but difficult. In one instance, a violinist I saw who had developed dystonia of the fourth and fifth fingers of the left hand was offered biomechanical retraining, but instead chose to switch his career to conducting. This is yet another positive way of coping. This actually happened to Robert Schumann, a brilliant pianist of the nineteenth century who became a conductor and composer after struggling with his loss of finger control. In his desperate attempt for a solution he created devices with springs and rubber bands as well as engaging in futile exercises that only seemed to make things worse.

Pianists seem to be the most frequent victims of focal dystonia, although this may be because it is the most frequently played instrument. It was the technique of one famous pianist that resulted in her injury. She had very long fingers that played in a flat, extended position. Other awkward positions also were part of her technique. Over time she developed a dystonia of the fourth and fifth fingers of the right hand, which would curve inward as she played, causing her to lose control. Poor technique is more likely to occur in less experienced pianists but also can occur in seasoned professionals. Sometimes the poor technique of a child prodigy, which the teacher might be afraid to correct, can result in injury later.

This pianist realized she could no longer play the dramatic romantic pieces in her repertoire and regretfully retired from the concert stage. She became profoundly depressed and went into virtual seclusion for a number of years. Desperate, she sought the help of medical professionals, all of whom agreed on the diagnosis of focal dystonia, but offered no definitive help. Undaunted, she searched for someone who might offer some retraining help. She finally found a teacher who specialized in the retraining of injured musicians and who set about modifying her technique. One of the first things the teacher suggested was changing her repertoire. He moved her on to music that was simpler, avoiding complex chords and scales. Gradually, with training exercises, she slowly began to improve. She was then taught additional tricks, such as slowing her pace and using her left hand to compensate for notes that her fourth and fifth fingers could no longer reach. She was also shown that by extending and holding the fourth and fifth fingers, followed by twisting the wrists and coming down on the keys in this fashion, some function of these fingers was possible. Her physician suggested that a certain surgical procedure also might be helpful. Here the plan was to sever the fibrous connection between the extensor tendons of the fourth and fifth fingers. It had been noted that when either of these fingers was flexed, it would pull the other finger down with it. The operation, a simple one, was performed and gave the pianist slightly more freedom, since now it was only the fifth finger that curled under because of the dystonia. After several years of hard, painstaking work, the pianist was able to return to the stage. In this case, sheer will and determination allowed this person to at least partly conquer a devastating illness.

Clarinet, Oboe, French Horn, Trumpet, and Bassoon

Clarinets and oboes are ergonomic nightmares. This is primarily because these instruments hang on a thumb hook, which upsets the total dynamic of finger action, especially if it is improperly placed. Ideally the clarinet or oboe should be unloaded from the thumb. Dr. H. J. H. Fry, a hand surgeon in Australia, has designed a neck strap and shoulder harness that, when coupled with a post that rests between the instrument and the chest, removes the need for a thumb rest. If a thumb rest is used, then the thumb should be in an anatomically comfortable position and the key lengths should be modified so that slightly curved fingers come comfortably into contact with the keys. The oboe has additional ergonomic problems for musicians who create their own reeds. This additional forearm and finger work can contribute to the development of RSI. The high pressures created in the oral cavity when playing the oboe have been reported to cause soft-palate paralysis.

Another ergonomic burden of the double reed player is the process of making reeds. Although reeds can by purchased ready-made, many professionals prefer to make their own. Reeds are made from a bamboolike cane called apundo donax. The cane is slit lengthwise in three pieces. This is followed by a meticulous set of steps that place great strain on the fingers, hands, and forearms. These steps include gouging and shaping the cane with a razor, tying it to a tube, and hoping it will produce a pure tone. Obviously, the injured oboist will have to find alternatives to making his or her own reeds.

Ergonomic principles apply to the French horn, where the levers are often not long enough. Soldering extensions to the levers can alleviate this problem. On the left hand, the fifth-finger open ring may be improperly placed and should be correctly positioned for this finger. A knee holder consisting of a sponge attached to the thigh will prevent discomfort from the notch that the horn usually presses into the thigh.

Both French horn and trumpet players can sustain complete or partial tears of the muscles surrounding the mouth. This is often referred to as "the Satchmo syndrome," which is the result of playing the instrument for prolonged periods while hitting high notes. The French horn has a particularly narrow rim on the mouthpiece, which may need to be changed. Surgical repair is possible if long periods of rest do not cure it.

The bassoon is another instrument that can cause both right- and left-hand problems, requiring key modification. It can be played suspended or with a floor spike, although some bassoonists claim there is a loss of flexibility with the spike and prefer the shoulder strap.

Percussion

Most of the drummers and other percussionists (vibraphone, xylophone, etc.) get into difficulty for two principal reasons. First, they all play physically demanding instruments, and the musicians are often in poor shape and may develop low back problems. Second, they are gripping their sticks too tightly and using only their wrists instead of their whole arms and shoulders in an integrated fashion.

Problems in the Orchestra

Seating

Very little consideration is given to proper seating for orchestra musicians or, for that matter, nonorchestra players such as the soloist. This is compounded by the fact that orchestras often travel, and seating varies in different halls. Seating should be stable, cushioned, and, ideally, suit the height of the musician.

Sound Control

Hearing problems are not an infrequent occurrence for orchestra as well as rock musicians. Attempts have been made to use plastic shields to protect certain orchestra musicians, but this is rarely done. Standard earplugs distort the nuances of sound that musicians need to hear to play in synchrony with others. A practical solution has been custom-fitting musicians with noise attenuators, specially fitted devices that are inserted in the ear and diminish the sound level but don't distort the quality of the music. All musicians should have periodic hearing tests.

Stage Fright

In a survey of over two thousand musicians conducted by the International Congress of Symphony and Orchestra Musicians (ICSOM), stage fright or performance anxiety was high on the list of health problems. Musicians have been known to cope with this by taking propanolol, a beta blocker, to quell their symptoms. It is advisable for musicians with this problem to seek professional advice.

Playing a musical instrument, although you might not have thought so, can be a dangerous profession. Evaluation of an injured musician proceeds along the same course as that of any other person with a work-related upper extremity disorder. In examining injured musicians, it is critical to observe them playing their respective instruments; videotaping is very helpful in this regard. Modifications of ergonomic and biomechanical factors are extremely important with musical injuries. Therapy proceeds along the same lines as for any RSI patient.

13

Other Causes
of RSI

A multitude of causes unknown to former times are now
acting with a combined force to blunt the discriminating
powers.

–William Wordsworth (1770–1850)

In addition to those already mentioned, many other work-
related upper extremity activities can lead to RSI. Although the
sources of injury may differ, RSI is a common final pathway. In
many cases these activities are carried out in addition to other
repetitive functions, such as computer use. The complaints in
this group are like those of many other RSI sufferers. The cul-
prits are similar: repetition, sustained activity, awkward positioning, deconditioned state, poor ergonomics. The following
examples by no means complete the roster of risky professions
but will give some idea of the range of professions at risk.

RSI and Court Stenographers

Anyone who has been to court or seen TV or movie court
scenes has noticed the ever-present court stenographer busily

working at a small machine near the judge's bench. As the operator plies the keys of the machine, a sheaf of encoded paper pops up and drops into a box at the back of the machine. Later this will be decoded and turned into court testimony. At one time, court reporting was done by hand. The stenograph machine was invented to increase speed, and was first used and gradually perfected in the late 1800s. An alternate version was developed for office secretaries taking dictation. As we have seen with the typewriter and computer, improvements were made not so much for comfort as for efficiency. This type of phonetic shorthand enabled the user to record 200 to 225 words per minute, more than double the speed obtainable with a typewriter. Stenograph machines as presently used come in several models, including one that can connect to a computer to provide a real-time transcription of testimony.

All of these machines have a similar setup consisting of twenty-five keys: thirteen of them for consonants and four for vowels. A syllable can be recorded with a single stroke. The fingers of the left hand generally type the beginning sound, which is usually a consonant, while the thumbs hit vowel keys. The right hand can type the syllable's end sound. Repetitive strain injury is not an uncommon result of this work.

Ergonomically, these machines are usually placed horizontally on a stand, causing the operator to keep the wrists in extension. One of the ergonomic modifications suggested is to secure an adjustable stand, now available, that allows the machine to be tilted downward, away from the operator so that the wrists are in a neutral position. The most comfortable posture for the operator is to straddle the machine so it is approached central to the body.

As I looked through some of the manuals for older stenograph machines, I found instructions for a "ladylike" posture for women. They were advised to position themselves sideways. This would cause their bodies and necks to be twisted to the right or left, a recipe for muscle imbalance leading to neck and shoulder problems. Even if such positioning is avoided, operation of the stenograph machine encourages the same kind of eventual postural misalignment seen with computer users or pianists. Posture deteriorates over time. The keys of the steno-graph machine have a soft touch but require more use of the thumbs than the typewriter or computer keyboard, where thumb use is generally limited to the space bar.

The court stenographer is also often asked to work over sus-tained periods of time, increasing the risk of injury. Very few stenograph users consider that they are engaged in an athletic activity that requires postural training and strengthening exercises to avoid injury. We have had to retrain a number of court stenog-raphers to modify their technique. A neutral wrist position and slightly curved fingers with short nails are part of this process. In addition, the stenographer may need to lighten his or her touch.

Court stenographers often work long hours in the courtroom but then must later transpose the phonetic coding into court tes-timony using a computer. Many of these people are in chronic pain and risk partial or permanent disability. While serving as an expert witness, I have been approached many times in the court-room by individual stenographers who were having their own problems with RSI. I have also testified for several court stenog-raphers at workers' compensation hearings. A few of my court stenographer patients, despite our best efforts, have had to leave what for them was a lucrative but punishing profession.

RSI in Garment Workers

Dr. Robert Harrison, clinical professor of medicine at the Uni-versity of California in San Francisco, and Jacqueline Chan, M.S., M.P.H., of the California Department of Health Service, have studied this population and created a model partnership between health services and worker advocates. Their goal was to lessen injury in a major industrial area. Worldwide clothing production is approximately a $335 billion business. Seventy-five percent of 11 million workers are women, about 793,000 of whom work in the United States. Dr. Harrison has described the main problems seen in these workers. They include generally unsafe conditions in many unlicensed shops, long hours with few breaks, no benefits, no control over work, cultural and language barriers, and workers' fear about reporting injury. All of these factors point to a high likelihood of injury. Indeed, sewing machine operators have significantly more symptoms of musculoskeletal distress than other garment workers. In one study of six shops, 91.9 percent of operators experienced symptoms. Eighty-seven percent complained of neck pain, 75 percent reported symptoms in the back and hips, 35 percent complained of pain in the hands and wrists, 35 percent noted pain in the legs, and 28 percent had pain in the arms and elbows.

The ergonomic problems faced by these workers included nonadjustable chairs, being forced to work in various awkward postures, repetitive pinching to push cloth through the machine, contact stress from pedals and levers, the requirement for a rapid pace of work, and no rotation of tasks. Some of the ergonomic solutions include table extensions with teacup holders, improved foot support, adjustable chairs with wedge and lumbar supports, and knee pedal cushions.

Because injuries among garment workers can be severe, patient care interventions were developed in the California project. These included a free clinic, clinical exams, physical therapy, massage and exercise classes, and ergonomic instruction.

Unfortunately, the relation of their work to their injury is generally not understood by these workers. Fear of job loss and a feeling that pain is an integral part of the job are also factors that thwart recovery.

Injuries among Dental Practitioners and Dental Surgeons

Dentists and dental practitioners are in a high-risk profession for RSI and are often the victims of severe injury. The same kinds of problems are encountered by certain medical specialists, including surgeons and ophthalmologists (see chapter 11), who often are forced to work in awkward positions performing fine, demanding work using the arms and fingers. According to Dr.

Robert Goldberg, associate clinical professor of occupational and environmental medicine at the University of California in San Francisco, risk factors in this field involve posture, upper extremity positioning, grip, repetition, force, and vibration. Injuries can be severe, so that the same rules of prevention we have discussed related to body conditioning and strengthening apply here.

Some of Dr. Goldberg's suggestions include the following:

- Patient positioning is important. While the typical patient position is slightly higher than horizontal, it would be better to place the patient in the full horizontal position, so that the practitioner is perpendicular to his or her patient and does not have to reach over the patient from an awkward position. In this fashion the practitioner can sit comfortably with good back support in an adjustable chair with feet firmly planted on the ground.

- Chair height should be adjusted so it is neither too low, forcing the practitioner to bend over the patient, or too high, putting him or her in a cramped posture with a twisted neck. The alignment of the practitioner is also important. Sitting "sidesaddle" and twisting the body while working produces gross misalignment of the body.

- Proper alignment results in the practitioner gaining full back support from the chair with feet firmly planted on the ground in straight body alignment. Footrests can be helpful in attaining good alignment. Another useful intervention is a magnifying loupe, which keeps the practitioner from crouching over and encourages good posture.

- Instrument use, design, and balance are important. When possible, instruments should be held with the wrist in a neutral position. As with writing instruments, increased barrel width can be more comfortable. When instruments are attached to a cord, the length should be such that the practitioner doesn't fight the cord while working. Finally, gloves that are too tight can hamper hand activity and cause fatigue. Although these are general suggestions, each practitioner armed with basic ergonomic information needs to adjust the workstation according to individual body measurements and space type of work.

Sign Language Interpreters

Sign language interpreting is known as a high-risk occupation for RSI. Patients I have seen can become seriously injured with a variety of upper body disorders similar to what might be seen with computer users or other persons engaged in repetitive activity.

Signing is a physically and mentally demanding profession. Following an intensive and difficult course of training, interpreters submit to an examination to be certified by the National Association of the Deaf (NAD). They may also gain and submit to a code of ethics promoted by the Registry of Interpreters for the Deaf (RID). Some work through agencies, while others freelance. Similar certification organizations exist in many countries of the world.

Sign language interpreters are under constant stress as they work. They must have a high level of awareness as they strive for absolute accuracy. Like the computer user, whose very art of sitting at the keyboard may cause the body to tense, the interpreter tends to tighten his or her entire body when beginning to work. The various positions of the hands and arms include vigorous use of the fingers and forearms in particular.

The hand is opened and closed rapidly. This is combined with supination and pronation at the elbow, ulnar deviation, radial deviation, extension, and flexion of the wrist. If the forearm and hand muscles are held tightly, then muscle groups will tend to work against each other and injury will occur. The head of the signer is often thrust forward and the shoulders and neck are held tightly, which can lead to the familiar findings of postural misalignment possibly leading to neurogenic thoracic outlet syndrome.

Good ergonomic rules for the signer will often depend on

the preparations made by those requesting the service. The sign language interpreter would do well to discuss these issues before beginning work. The signer should be provided with a good straight-back chair without armrests. When the signer is seated and working, there should be no obstruction between him or her and the target audience. Good lighting is essential. In the case of a slide show or theater presentation, the signer should be in the beam of a spotlight, and any glare from open windows or direct sunlight should be eliminated.

Biomechanical retraining may be necessary to allow the signer to move in a more relaxed fashion, avoiding exaggerated or excessive motion. Stretching and strengthening upper body muscles are critical to protect against injury. Signers should not work more than one-half to three-quarters of an hour at a stretch without a break. If the session is more than one and one-half hours, an alternate signer to assist would be necessary. Various sign language organizations specify the work limitations in their work protocols.

There are, of course, a whole host of other professions where upper body injuries can occur. Think of the artist, the butcher, the poultry worker, or the cook. A fisherman from Alaska who injured himself cutting the heads off salmon recently wrote to me. Similar injuries often occur in these different professions and should be treated similarly. The keys, as we have indicated, are a complete physical exam done by a knowledgeable provider, followed by biomechanical and ergonomic intervention under the supervision of a qualified physical or occupational therapist. A continuing conditioning program completes the picture for all upper body workers.

14

Beating RSI: A Five-Step Protection Plan

Wouldn't it be great if you could avoid suffering from RSI for life? It can happen if you take the knowledge you've gained reading this book and put it into action. There are obstacles to overcome even if you've undergone successful treatment. Relapses are not uncommon, especially if you revert to your old ways of doing things. These can be minimized and eventually eliminated as you learn how to cope with the illness. Keep in mind that with RSI you are recovering, not necessarily recovered. What follows is an outline of the steps you need to follow toward your goal of beating RSI for life. It won't be easy, but it is certainly worth the effort.

Step 1: Examine Your Life

Assess your risk for injury by taking a good look at your activities both at work and elsewhere. You might find it useful to write down each of your daily activities, along with time spent and degree of intensity. The list can give you a good idea of your risk profile. Think about what's going on in your life every day and ask yourself questions: Does your boss subject you to long hours, short deadlines, and binge work? Do you do this to yourself? Do you work more than two to four hours at a time at a computer? Do you use a mouse, laptop, phone, or other equipment intensely? Even pushing and pulling on filing cabinets can lead to backaches and postural problems and can contribute to RSI. Are your chair, workstation, and other equipment sources of obvious discomfort? Is your life full of enormous repetitive chores and responsibilities that put you under stress? Are you having trouble sleeping or eating? Has your work affected your sex life? Do you feel depressed?

In doing this self-assessment, don't forget to recognize the potential for injury from what you do when you are at home. While such activities may be a symptom of injury, they can also contribute to your problem. Dusting, vacuuming, washing floors and dishes, gardening, and writing can all tip you over the edge. Certain sports can contribute to injury. Golf, tennis, basketball, and skiing can all enhance risk of injury.

If you think about these factors as you examine your list, you may notice that you are doing too much. This self-appraisal is the first step in helping you become informed about what is necessary to reach your goal.

Step 2: Get a Physical Evaluation

Self-evaluation is difficult and not as objective as the opinion of a qualified professional, who may detect things you don't know you have. To start, learn something about how you are put together. I've tried to help with this by discussing some anatomy in chapter 1. This will enable you to understand what the physician or therapist is doing. You'll know why you are receiving certain medications or which group of muscles needs work and why. Although RSI is sometimes described as a musculoskeletal illness, it also involves nerves, muscles, tendons, ligaments, and vascular structures. Taking the trouble to learn about your own anatomy will help you understand how that information relates to other steps in this program.

Physical and occupational therapists are trained to evaluate your musculoskeletal system. They have to be able to do this to correct specific problem areas. First they would look for derangement of posture. If you have been working for years slumped over a desk, your posture is bound to deteriorate. These changes mark the beginning of a continuing process that can eventually result in RSI even before age thirty. The people I usually see in my practice are relatively young, otherwise healthy, but nevertheless disabled. This paradox of a healthy-looking patient with severe physical limitations is one cause of the abundant skepticism of health care professionals. Certain illnesses, such as type II diabetes and obesity, need to be ruled out as contributing causes. Recent research has shown that osteoarthritis may be related to long-standing RSI. One theory is that tightened muscles place extra strain on joints or tendons, producing wear and tear.

Step 3. Plan Prevention and Cure

Assuming you now have some basic knowledge about where you stand, the next step is to begin to take proper care of your body either to prevent injury or to care for an existing injury. These measures have to include taking care of workstation deficiencies, problems at home, and other issues relating to your physical activities.

Once you have found the right treatment team, you can begin working with the physical or occupational therapist, who can guide you in a carefully orchestrated program of stretches and exercises. These are outlined in chapter 7. Now your job is to do the stretches and exercises at home under the guidance of your therapist. I can't overemphasize the importance of continuity and consistency in performing exercises and stretches on your own. This is where people who have improved get hung up—they stop the exercises because they think they don't need to do them anymore, or because they're simply bored with them. If you become too busy to do them, this may be a sign that you are headed for a relapse. Daily exercise accomplishes several things. It enables you to defeat the process of postural deterioration, which progresses insidiously over time and leads to RSI. Stretching and strengthening muscles improve blood supply to all soft tissues, the key to both avoiding relapse and preventing problems to begin with. The neuromuscular therapeutic program will emphasize upper body work, but you shouldn't neglect the condition of your lower back and extremities. Problems below can affect the upper body, too, because muscles that are deconditioned can affect the function of muscles elsewhere. These concepts are discussed in chapters 7 and 11.

If you are having a hard time getting started because of advanced or painful injury, you also may need pain medication. This will allow the therapist to work on your soft tissues and allow you to get started cautiously with your exercises. If you are depressed you may need medicine, and some antidepressants also are helpful in controlling pain (see chapter 5). A psychiatric evaluation is advisable. Once you begin this process, you're on your way to both treating your RSI and diminishing the likelihood of relapse. The next step involves applying your knowledge of ergonomics to what you do.

Step 4: Pay Attention to Ergonomics

Fit the equipment to yourself, not yourself to the equipment. We should not be made to put ourselves in awkward positions to accommodate the instruments we work with. It is critical to embrace this concept because it will add to the likelihood that your recovery and RSI prevention will be permanent.

Changes you make in your workstation or your musical instrument can play an extremely important role in keeping you out of trouble. They may even be enough to make a dramatic impact on recovery. This may require investing in new equipment, such as a chair, pullout tray, keyboard, or mouse. Musicians might have to modify their instruments or make other positional changes. We have looked at some of these issues in chapter 11. By doing this you've added an additional layer of protection against injury.

Another important component of ergonomics is what might be called intrinsic ergonomics or biomechanics—the ways in which you use your body to perform work tasks. To correct biomechanical deficiencies that, because of awkward positioning, place a strain on soft tissues may require the help of a specialist in interpreting and eliminating incorrect movement patterns. The trick is to use your body efficiently—in essence, getting more miles to the gallon. Many, but not all, physical and occupational therapists are adept at evaluating movement. If you can find someone skilled in this area, it can be very helpful.

Step 5: Work the Health Care System

Whether you work for a company that provides insurance or carry your own policy, you may find it hard to get payment for the help and attention you need. A work-related injury usually puts you under the care of a workers' compensation carrier. Workers' compensation insurance benefits vary from state to state, and dealing with the bureaucracy can be onerous. As a result, many people choose not to get involved unless the injury is very serious. A recent study reported that only 11 percent of workers actually used workers' compensation for an injury. Most simply did not seek care or preferred to use their own care provider. Finding the right health care providers who understand RSI is not easy. The subjective nature of your pain and other symptoms can lead to skepticism and resentment by your employer, fellow workers, your physician, and your insurance carrier. This is the most frustrating part of the battle for care and attention. Of the patients I have seen, about 60 percent were still working despite pain and other symptoms. If you have to work under these conditions it can lead to a progression of symptoms and condemn you to an uncomfortable and stressful life.

One of my patients who was a financial translator in a bank was pushed to the limit by her employer because her skills were unique. Eventually she became seriously injured and was forced to leave her job. She came to see me, and after her diagnosis was given an exercise and stretching program for her repetitive strain injuries, which included neck mobility problems relating to thoracic outlet syndrome as well as postural misalignment. Seen in a normal social situation, it would be difficult to determine that she was ill. She continued to exercise and stretch but could not get the sustained and progressive input of her physical therapist because her insurance company cut off her benefits despite the fact that she was unable to work a full day. Her employer had no alternate position for her. She pursued her attempts to reinstate her benefits. After much travail she obtained a disability award. Soon afterward, however, she had to face an appeal by her insurance carrier which included seeing an "independent" medical examiner, who concluded that he doubted the existence of her disability. This sort of frustration and uncertainty is not uncommon and is a great source of stress.

It is difficult to obtain an effective answer to this problem except to urge patients to continue to fight for their rights. You may need the help of a lawyer or other professional to advocate for you.

What else can you do to make it easier to prevent RSI or improve your condition? Remember that you are essentially an athlete who has to remain in shape to work safely. Weight loss, proper diet, exercise, stretches, recreation, and rest breaks can all help you successfully manage your RSI program. Doing these things consistently for a lifetime is really a challenge, but it's certainly worth the effort.

Glossary

acupuncture The Chinese method of inserting needles into specific areas of the body to relieve pain.

acupressure The process of pressing specific areas of the body to relieve pain.

accommodation The ability of the lens of the eye to adjust for various distances; this ability diminishes with age.

acuity The clarity or clearness of vision.

Adson's test This is used to determine the presence of blood vessel compression in thoracic outlet syndrome by placing the head in specific positions to see if pulses are lost or diminished.

Allen test A clinical test for blockage of the ulnar artery or radial arteries at the wrist.

allodynia Occurs when a stimulus such as mechanical pressure produces pain when there should be none.

alpha receptors Alpha adrenergic receptors respond to adrenaline (norepinephrine) and certain blocking agents.

ANA *See* antinuclear antibody.

anomaly An abnormal anatomic structure not typically present.

antidepressants A group of medications used to treat depression and other psychological problems. Two principal groups are the tricyclics and the selective serotonin reuptake inhibitors (SSRIs).

antinuclear antibody (ANA) A lab test used for the detection of various connective tissue diseases such as lupus.

anxiety   An unpleasant emotional state that is an anticipation of real or imagined danger.

arcade of Fröhse   A fibrous tunnel that is a portion of the supinator muscle at the elbow. Present in 30 percent of adults, it is implicated in the compression of the radial nerve (radial tunnel syndrome).

autonomic dysfunction   Abnormality in the involuntary or autonomic nervous system. A common finding in persons with RSI on physical examination.

autonomic nervous system (sympathetic and parasympathetic nervous system)   The portion of the nervous system concerned with regulating cardiac muscle, smooth muscle, and glands that are not under your direct control.

binocularity   The ability of the eyes to fuse images and create one three-dimensional image.

biomechanics   The application of mechanical laws to living structures. It is the investigation of how we move.

brachial plexopathy   *See* brachial plexus or thoracic outlet syndrome.

brachial plexus   A network of nerves that unite in the neck area, tying the front portion of the last four cervical nerves to most of the first thoracic spinal nerves (see figure 15). The brachial plexus forms several branches as it leaves the neck. Compression of the brachial plexus or its branches is called brachial plexopathy or neurogenic thoracic outlet syndrome.

bone scan   A technique using radioisotopes to detect abnormalities in bony tissue.

calcium channel   A protein channel that is permeable to calcium and sodium ions that are found in cells. Calcium channel blockers are used in the treatment of hypertension.

carpal tunnel syndrome   Median nerve compression at the wrist often associated with repetitive motion and other causes.

carrying angle   The fixed angle at the elbow between the humerus and the ulna bones. Women tend to have larger carrying angles than men do.

causalgia   *See* complex regional pain syndrome (CRPS).

CTD   *See* cumulative trauma disorders.

cervical radiculopathy   A disease of the root of a spinal nerve, especially that portion of the root between the spinal cord and the vertebra that forms the canal that the spinal nerve passes through.

clavicle (collar bone)   Combined with the first rib, it forms a tight space where brachial plexus nerve compression can occur.

complex regional pain syndrome (CRPS)   A painful immobilizing syndrome linked to the sympathetic nervous system, of which there are two types: Type 1, formerly RSD, and Type 2, formerly causalgia. Symptoms of both types are similar and consist of burning pain, swelling, stiffness, and skin and bone changes in its later stages.

computer vision syndrome (CVS)   Eye problems relating to the use of the computer such as dry eyes, eye strain, headache, and blurred vision.

computerized tomography (CT scan)   A computer-assisted X-ray technique that increases clarity and decreases radiation exposure.

concentric contraction   Muscle contraction in which tension in the muscle is greater than the external load on the muscle, resulting in muscle shortening.

COX-1 and COX-2   *See* cyclooxygenase systems.

CT scan   *See* computerized tomography.

cubital tunnel syndrome   Results from injury, compression, or traction of the ulnar nerve at the elbow resulting in pain, numbness, and weakness of the forearm and hand. It is commonly found in RSI.

cumulative trauma disorders (CTDs)   One of many synonyms for RSI.

CVS   *See* computer vision syndrome.

cyclooxygenase systems (COX-1 and COX-2)   Enzymes found in tissues that have homeostatic functions (COX-1) and result from inflammation in tissues (COX-2). Inhibition of COX-2 enzymes is desirable, while inhibition of COX-1 enzymes is not. Certain enzymes affect either or both of these systems.

deep tendon reflexes (DTRs or tendon jerks)   The involuntary contractions of muscles after brief stretching, caused by tapping of the muscle's tendons.

Dellon's test   *See* two-point discrimination test.

DeQuervain's disease   A painful inflammation due to friction and tightness of the common tendon sheath of the abductor pollicis longus muscle and the extensor pollicis brevis muscles at the base of the thumb.

depression   A state of depressed mood characterized by feelings of sadness, despair, and discouragement. Often accompanied by feelings of low self-esteem, guilt, and eating and sleep disturbances.

dorsiflexion   Flexion or bending of a limb toward the extensor surface (flexing upward as in pushing a door).

Double-jointedness   *See* hyperlaxity.

Dupuytren's contracture   Flexion deformity of the fingers due to fibrosis of the palmar fascia (the covering of the palmar hand muscles).

dynamometer   Device for measuring force or strength, such as grip or pinch dynamometers.

EAST (elevated arm stress test)   *See* Roos test.

eccentric contraction   This occurs when an already stretched muscle contracts while in use. Excessive eccentric muscle contraction in an elongated muscle can be damaging to that muscle.

electroneurography (NVC)   A technique used to measure the conduction, velocity, and latency of peripheral nerves. Considered the "gold standard" for diagnosing carpal tunnel syndrome.

electromyogram (EMG)   A technique used to measure the duration and intensity of muscle activity. Usually done in conjunction with electroneurography.

EMG   *See* electromyogram.

epicondyle   A normal bump on a bone where tendons are attached to the bone.

epicondylitis   Inflammation of the epicondyle and its adjacent tendon.

ergonomics   The science of relating man to his work, applying anatomic, physiologic, and mechanical principles to produce efficiency in the work.

eustress   Mental, emotional, or physical stimuli that result in pleasure.

eye dominance   The eye that is used predominantly in the visual process. It does not necessarily correlate to hand dominance.

fibromyalgia   Characterized by widespread muscle pain not usually associated with weakness. A number of other symptoms, including joint pain, headache, and gastrointestinal symptoms, may also be present. Multiple painful trigger points are helpful in making the diagnosis. It occurs predominantly in women.

fibrosis   The replacement of normal tissue by fibrous scar tissue at the site of injury.

Finkelstein's test   In this test, one makes a fist with the thumb underneath the fingers and moves the fist in the direction of the fifth finger in ulnar deviation. If there is pain at the base of the thumb, DeQuervain's tenosynovitis is present.

flicker   The flickering movement of a CRT computer image based on the refresh or scanning rate of the picture.

foramen   A natural opening through bone or soft tissue.

ganglion cyst   The most common swelling in the hand, which usually arises from the tendon sheath and is often found on the dorsum (top) of the wrist.

gamekeeper's thumb   *See* ulnar collateral ligament tear.

golfer's elbow   *See* medial epicondylitis.

glucose (dextrose)   Sugar in fruits, plants, and in the blood of all animals. Blood glucose is elevated in diabetes mellitus.

grip strength   In this test one makes a fist while holding a grip dynamometer, and the quantity of the force generated is measured.

Guyon's canal syndrome (ulnar tunnel syndrome)   Ulnar nerve compression at the wrist occurring in the ulnar tunnel, which is made up of the pisiform and hamate bones on each side of the nerve and roofed over by the transverse carpal ligament.

humerus   The upper arm bone, which connects above with the scapula and below with the radius and ulna bones.

hyperlaxity   The ability of a joint to move beyond the normal range of motion of most people. Also called double-jointedness.

intrinsic muscles of the hand   A group of muscles that move the fingers and thumb in many directions. They consist of the interossei and lumbricals as well as the abductor pollicis brevis, opponens pollicis, flexor pollicis brevis, abductor pollicis, adductor pollicis, palmaris brevis, abductor digiti quinti, flexor digiti quinti brevis, and opponens digiti quinti. They mostly act as a group to provide the sophisticated movement necessary for the hand.

iontophoresis   The induction by means of an electric current of ions of soluble salts and medicines into the tissues as a means of introducing these medicines into the body.

isometric contraction   Muscle contraction in which tension of the muscle equals the external load on the muscle, resulting in constant muscle length.

isotonic contraction   Muscle contraction in which a constant internal tension is developed, resulting in a concentric muscle contraction.

lateral epicondylitis (tennis elbow)   Inflammation of the bony eminence at the elbow from which the wrist extensor muscle tendons originate.

ligament   A band of fibrous tissue that connects bones or cartilage and that supports and strengthens joints.

Linburg's anomalous tendon   Fibrous or tendinous bands connecting the flexor pollicis longus and index profundus tendons. An anomaly that restricts independent thumb flexion when the index finger is extended.

magnetic resonance imaging   A noninvasive diagnostic technique used to image the structure of the body. The patient is placed in the field of an electromagnet capable of producing images in a variety of planes. It is used primarily to evaluate soft tissues. The procedure is considered to be without risk to the patient except under certain circumstances.

MSDs   *See* musculoskeletal disorders.

mechanical allodynia   The result of pressure on soft tissues that produces pain that normally would not occur.

medial epicondylitis (golfer's elbow)   Inflammation of the bony eminence at the elbow from which the wrist flexor forearm pronator groups of muscles originate.

MRI   *See* magnetic resonance imaging.

musculoskeletal disorders (MSDs)   A term used to described the variety of symptoms caused by repetitive motion.

myofascial pain syndrome   Muscle pain and soreness often associated with repetitive motion.

nerve conduction velocity (NCV)   *See* electroneurography.

NSAIDs   *See* nonsteroidal anti-inflammatory drugs.

nociceptors   Nerve fibers responsible for the sensation of pain.

nonsteroidal anti-inflammatory drugs (NSAIDs)   A group of compounds with similar analgesic and anti-inflammatory properties; now divided into conventional and gastrointestinal protective.

norepinephrine   A naturally occurring catecholamine that is a major neurotransmitter released in response to stress and hypotension (lowered blood pressure).

occupational overuse syndrome (OOS)   One of many synonyms for repetitive strain injury (RSI).

overuse syndrome   A synonym for repetitive strain injury usually applied to musicians' injuries.

panic disorder   A state of extreme anxiety associated with disorganization of personality and function.

paresthesias   Abnormal sensations of tingling and numbness.

phonophoresis   The induction of medication into the tissues using high-frequency sound waves.

Physioball (Resistaball)   An inflatable plastic ball that comes in different sizes; useful for stretching and other exercises.

pinch test   In this test using a pinch dynamometer, three pinch strengths are tested. Pulp pinch (like the way one holds a sheet of paper), key pinch (like one grips a key), and chuck grip (like the grip on a pencil with thumb below and forefinger and middle finger above) are measured by exerting pressure on the dynamometer.

postural misalignment   In RSI, a term used to describe a typical round-shouldered, head-forward posture that is a key factor in causing soft tissue nerve traction and compression problems related to pain, discomfort, and other symptoms. Postural misalignment is also often associated with scoliosis and lordosis and is the most common finding in persons with RSI.

pronation   Position of the palm downward, as in typing.

pronator teres muscle syndrome   Compression of the median nerve in the forearm as a result of compression by the pronator teres muscle.

proprioception   The conduction of sensory nerve signals that indicate muscle and joint position to the central nervous system.

prostaglandins   Potent mediators of a diverse group of physiologic processes. PGE2 is an important prostaglandin, which increases vascular permeability, increases pain sensitivity, and raises temperature. NSAIDs and aspirin inhibit prostaglandin activity.

radial deviation   Position of the hand in the direction of the radial bone on the thumb side of the hand. The opposite of ulnar deviation.

radial tunnel syndrome   Compression of the radial nerve as it passes under the tendinous arch of the supinator muscle at the elbow.

radius   The bone on the outer or thumb side of the forearm. It articulates above with the humerus and the ulna and below with the ulna and the wrist bones.

Raynaud's syndrome   A painful condition affecting the fingers or toes caused by compromised circulation and provoked by cold. The digits turn white for lack of blood supply.

reflex sympathetic dystrophy (RSD)   *See* complex regional pain syndrome (CRPS).

reflex sympathetic dysfunction   Overactivity of the involuntary sympathetic nervous system causing temperature and color changes as well as sweating in the extremities.

regional arm pain   A term used by some to describe the pain associated with RSI.

REM sleep   A term used to describe the rapid eye movement phase of sleep.

Resistaball   *See* Physioball.

Roos test   A test done with arms in the air, in the "hold up" position, to see how long the position can be sustained without producing pain, numbness, or color changes in the skin for a three-minute limit. It is an important clinical test in the diagnosis of thoracic outlet syndrome. See also EAST test.

rotator cuff   A musculotendinous structure of the shoulder joint formed by the linked fibers of the supraspinatus, infraspinatus, teres minor, and subscapularis muscles giving the shoulder stability, exceptional range of motion, and strength.

satellite cell   A mononuclear stem cell found between the muscle fiber and its surrounding basal lamina. When activated it initiates the first phase of muscle fiber regeneration.

scalene bands   Anomalous fibrous connections between scalene muscles, sometimes resulting in brachial plexus nerve impairment.

scalene muscles   Muscles on either side of the neck composed of three sections that raise the ribs, rotate the neck, and bend and flex the spine. The anterior and median muscles can squeeze the nerves of the brachial plexus, causing the more common form of thoracic outlet syndrome.

Semmes-Weinstein test   The application of threadlike fibers of varying thickness to evaluate sensory nerves in the hands.

sodium channel   A protein channel in cells; selective for the passage of sodium ions.

splints   A rigid or flexible appliance used to immobilize or protect an injured part of the body.

stress   Usually defined as the sum of biologic reactions to mental, emotional, or physical stimuli that tend to disturb the homeostasis of the body and that may lead to certain disorders.

supination   Turning the palm upward.

supinator syndrome   *See* radial tunnel syndrome.

TENS (transcutaneous electrical nerve stimulator)   An electrical device that stimulates nerve fibers that travel to the brain and that produces relief of pain.

tendinitis   Inflammation of tendons or their attachment to muscle.

tendon   A fibrous cord attached to muscle or bone that conveys the action of the muscle to the joint.

tendon sheath   A tunnel or sheath that guides a tendon around a curve; analogous to the ring on a fishing rod.

tennis elbow   *See* lateral epicondylitis.

tenosynovitis   Inflammation of the tendon sheath (e.g., DeQuervain's tenosynovitis).

TFCC   *See* triangulate fibrocartilage complex.

thermography (thermal video camera, computer-assisted thermography)   A technique using an infrared camera to photographically portray body surface temperature.

Tinel's sign   This test is performed by lightly tapping along the line of a nerve. If tingling is felt, the test is positive for nerve impairment.

thoracic outlet syndrome (TOS)   This is classified as neurogenic (95 percent) and vascular (5 percent). It is basically the result of compression of the brachial plexus nerve trunks or the subclavian artery or vein. The neurogenic type is quite common in RSI and appears to be due to soft-tissue compression of the nerves due to poor posture or anatomic anomalies.

transverse carpal ligament   A ligament that functions as a tendon pulley, which is the roof of the carpal and ulnar tunnels. It is surgically cut in carpal tunnel syndrome to relieve pressure on the carpal tunnel.

triangulate fibrocartilage complex (TFCC)   A complex structure that stabilizes the wrist. A cause of wrist pain when perforated. It is associated with wrist fractures and other injuries.

trapezius   A flat, triangular muscle covering the upper and back part of the neck and shoulders. It is divided into upper and lower portions. They rotate the scapula. The upper portion, alone, moves the scapula upward and braces the shoulder. The lower part, alone, drives the scapula downward.

trigger finger   A tendon entrapment involving the fingers or thumb. More common in women and characterized by locking of a nodule in the finger pulley associated with pain on flexion.

two-point discrimination test   A test used to predict functional nerve recovery. Two blunt points (a paperclip is typically used) are moved along the long axis of the limb or finger. The distance between the two points is decreased until the two points can no longer be distinguished.

UBE   *See* upper-body ergometer.

ulna   The inner large bone of the forearm opposite the thumb. Above, it articulates with the humerus and the radius, and below, with the wrist bones on the side of the fifth finger.

ulnar collateral ligament tear (gamekeeper's thumb)   When torn, the ulnar collateral ligament causes instability of the thumb. It can result from falling with an outstretched hand or tight gripping and twisting.

ulnar deviation   Position of the hand in the direction of the ulna bone. A common malpositioning in typists and pianists.

ulnar tunnel syndrome   *See* Guyon's canal syndrome.

upper-body ergometer (UBE)   An upper-body exercise device useful for increasing shoulder and arm range of motion and strength.

vertebra   One of thirty-three bones of the spinal column, including the cervical, thoracic, lumbar, sacral, and coccygeal sections.

Wartenberg's syndrome   An isolated neuritis of the superficial branch of the radial nerve at the wrist, especially caused by external compression such as wearing a splint or a tight watchband.

Wright's test   A one-minute test where arms are raised and held against the ears to evaluate compression and traction of the brachial plexus in thoracic outlet.

Further Reading

Introduction

Reid, J., C. Ewan, and E. Loy. 1991. Pilgrimage of pain: The illness experiences of women with repetitive strain injury and the search for credibility. *Social Science Medicine* 32:601–612.

Stevens, J. C., J. C. Witt, E. S. Benn, and A. L. Weaver. 2001. The frequency of carpal tunnel syndrome in computer users at a medical facility. *Neurology* 56:1568–1570.

U.S. Department of Labor. 1999. Occupational Safety and Health Administration, 29 CFR part 1910. Ergonomics program, proposed rule, part 22. November 23.

Chapter 1: Understanding RSI

Groopman, J. 2000. Hurting all over: With so many people in so much pain how could fibromyalgia not be a disease? *The New Yorker,* November 13.

Mackinnon, S. E., and C. B. Novak. 1997. Repetitive strain in the workplace. *Journal of Hand Surgery* 22 (1): 2–18.

Magee, D. J. 1987. *Orthopedic Physical Assessment.* New York: W. B. Saunders.

Pascarelli, E. F., and Y. P. Hsu. 2001. Understanding work-related upper extremity disorders: Clinical findings in 485 computer users, musicians, and others. *Journal of Occupational Rehabilitation* 11 (1): 1–21.

Chapter 2: Getting the Diagnosis

Beasley, R., N. Raymond, S. Hill, M. Nowitz, and R. Hughes. 2003. Venous thromboembolism in a computer user. *European Respiratory Journal* 21: 374–376.

Brooke, James. 2002. Youth let their thumbs do the talking in Japan. *New York Times,* May 9.

Gordon, S. L., S. J. Blair, and L. F. Fine, eds. 1995. *Repetitive Motion Disorders of the Upper Extremity.* Rosemont, Ill.: American Academy of Orthopedic Surgeons.

Machleder, H. I. 1998. Neurogenic thoracic outlet compression syndrome. In *Vascular Disorders of the Upper Extremity,* 3rd ed., ed. H. I. Machleder, 131–135. Mount Kisco, N.Y.: Futura.

Millender, L. H., ed. 1992. *Occupational Disorders of the Upper Extremity.* Livingstone, N.Y.: Churchill.

Pécina, M. M., J. Krmpotic-Nemanic, and A. D. Markiewitz. 1991. *Tunnel Syndromes.* Boca Raton, Fla.: CRC Press.

Roos, D. B. 1976. Congenital anomalies associated with thoracic outlet syndrome: Anatomy, symptoms, diagnosis, and treatment. *American Journal of Surgery* 132 (6): 771–778.

———. 1990. The thoracic outlet syndrome is underrated. *Archives of Neurology* 47 (3): 327–328.

Silverstein, B. A., D. S. Stetson, W. M. Keyserling, and L. J. Fine. 1997. Work-related musculoskeletal disorders: Comparison of data sources for surveillance. *American Journal of Industrial Medicine* 31 (5): 600–608.

Sjogaard, G, and B. R. Jensen. 1996. Muscle pathology with overuse. *Chronic Upper Limb Musculo-Skeletal Injuries in the Workplace,* ed. D. Ranney. Philadelphia: W. B. Saunders.

Sucher, B. M., and D. M. Heath. 1993. Thoracic outlet syndrome—a myofascial variant. Part 3: Structural and postural considerations. *Journal of the American Osteopathic Association* 93 (3): 334, 340–345.

Chapter 3: RSI and Your Emotions

Charney, D. S., and A. Deutch. 1996. A functional neuroanatomy of anxiety and fear: Implications for the pathophysiology and treatment of anxiety disorders. *Critical Review of Neurobiology* 10 (3–4): 419–446.

Friedman, T. L. 2000. Cyberserfdom. *New York Times,* July 30.

Raskin, N. H., M. W. Howard, and W. K. Ehrenfeld. 1985. Headache as the leading symptom of the thoracic outlet syndrome. *Headache* 25 (4): 208–210.

Reid, J., C. Ewan, and E. Lowy. 1991. Pilgrimage of pain: The illness experiences of women with repetitive strain injury and the search for credibility. *Social Science Medicine* 32: 601–612.

Sheon, R. P. 1997. Repetitive strain injury: An overview of the problem and the patients: The Gulf Group. *Postgraduate Med* 102 (4) 53–56, 62–68.

Tarkan, L. 2000. Athletes' injuries go beyond the physical. *New York Times,* September 26.

Tenner, E. 1996. *Why Things Bite Back: Technology and the Revenge of Unintended Consequences.* New York: Alfred A. Knopf.

Chapter 4: RSI and Your Eyes

Leavitt, S. B. 1995. *Vision Comfort at VDTs.* Glenview, Ill.: Leavitt Medical Communications.

Chapter 5: Managing Pain

Bombardier, C., L. Laine, A. Reicin, D. Shapiro, R. Burgos-Vargas, B. Davis, R. Day, et al. 2000. Comparison of upper gastrointestinal toxicity of rofecoxib and naproxen in patients with rheumatoid arthritis: VIGOR Study Group. *New England Journal of Medicine* 343 (21): 1520–1528.

FitzGerald, G. A., and C. Patrono. 2001. The coxibs, selective inhibitors of cyclooxygenase-2. *New England Journal of Medicine* 345(6):433–442.

Hooshman, H. 1993. Chronic pain. In *Reflex Sympathetic Dystrophy Prevention and Management,* 202. Boca Raton, Fla.: CRC Press.

Pittman, D. M., and M. J. Belgrade. 1997. Complex regional pain syndrome. *American Family Physician* 56 (9): 2265–2270, 2275–2276.

Victor, M., A. H. Ropper, R. D. Adams, and M. Victor. 2000. *Adams and Victor's Principles of Neurology,* 7th ed. New York: McGraw-Hill.

Chapter 6: Your Lower Back

Tulder, M., and B. W. van Koes. 2001. Low back pain and sciatica. *Clinical Evidence* 5:772–789.

Frymoyer, J. W. 1988. Back pain and sciatica. *New England Journal of Medicine* 318 (5): 291–300.

Snook, S. H., R. A. Campanelli, and J. W. Hart. 1978. A study of three preventive approaches to low back injury. *Journal of Occupational Medicine* 20 (7): 478–481.

Chapter 7: Physical and Occupational Therapy for RSI

Jordan, S. E., S. S. Ahn, J. A. Freisclag, H. A. Gelabert, and H. I. Machleder. 2000. Selective botulin chemodenervation of the scalene muscles for treatment of neurogenic thoracic outlet syndrome. *Annals of Vascular Surgery* 14 (4): 365–369.

Novak, C. B. 1996. Conservative management of thoracic outlet syndrome. *Seminars in Thoracic and Cardiovascular Surgery* 8 (2): 201–207.

Chapter 8: Ergonomics: Making Your Equipment Fit

Armstrong, T. J., L. J. Fine, S. A. Goldstein, Y. R. Lifshitz, and B. A. Silverstein. 1987. Ergonomics considerations in hand and wrist tendinitis. *Journal of Hand Surgery* 12 (5, pt. 2): 830–837.

Bommarito, P. F., M. R. Sandberg, and G. D. Shurts. 2001. Survey of laptop computers at Lawrence Livermore National Laboratory. Washington, D.C.: U.S. Department of Energy, UCRL-AR-146102.

Bruce, O., C. Dickerson, and C. Zenz, eds. 1994. *Occupational Medicine,* 3rd ed. St. Louis: C. V. Mosby.

Kay, M. 2003. "Type It Anywhere." *Scientific American,* January, 32–33.

Kroemer, K. H. E., and E. Grandjean. 1997. *Fitting the Task to the Human: A Textbook of Occupational Ergonomics,* 5th ed. London: Taylor & Francis.

Tenner, E. 1997. How the chair conquered the world. *Wilson Quarterly* Spring: 64–70.

Peper, E., and K. H. Gibney. 1997. Computer solutions to computer pain: How to stay healthy at the computer with e-mail tips BMVG. *Berkely Peachpit Press Newsletter* 13 (2): 174–175.

Chapter 9: Biomechanics: Using Your Body

Pascarelli, E. F. 1999. Training and retraining of office workers and musicians. *Occupational Medicine* 14 (1): iv, 163–172.

Pascarelli, E., and J. Kella. 1993. Soft-tissue injuries related to use of the computer keyboard: A clinical study of 53 severely injured persons. *Journal of Occupational Medicine* 35 (5): 522–532.

Chapter 10: At Home with RSI

The information in this chapter is from personal communications with Lisa Sattler, P.T., Vera Wills, and Yu-Pin Hsu, O.T.

Chapter 11: Getting Back to Work

Kanigel, R. 1996. Frederick Taylor's apprenticeship. *Wilson Quarterly* Summer: 44–51.

Morse, T., C. Dillon, and N. Warren. 2000. Reporting of work-related musculoskeletal disorder (MSD) to workers' compensation, 281–292. Amityville, N.Y.: New Solutions, Baywood Publishing.

Thompson, N. 2002. Make Mine DVORAK: One writer's love affair with the other keyboard layout. February 5. http://www.slate.msn.com/toolbar.aspx?action=print&id=2061547.

Chapter 12: RSI and Musicians

Diagram Group. 1976. *Musical Instruments of the World: An Illustrated Encyclopedia*. New York: Paddington Press.

Graffman, G. 1986. Doctor, can you lend an ear? *Medical Problems of Performing Artists* 1: 1–3.

Hsu, Yu-Pin. 1997. An analysis of contributing factors to repetitive strain injury (RSI) among pianists, 481–506. Ann Arbor, Mich.: UMI Dissertation Service.

Lederman, R. J. 1986. Thoracic Outlet Syndrome: Review of the controversies and a report of 17 instrumental musicians. *Medical Problems of Performing Artists* 2: 87.

Newmark, J., and F. H. Hochberg. 1987. Isolated painless manual incoordination in 57 musicians. *Journal of Neurology and Neurosurgical Psychiatry* 50 (3): 291–295.

Chapter 13: Other Causes of RSI

Feuerstein, M., and T. E. Fitzgerald. 1992. Biomechanical factors affecting upper extremity cumulative trauma disorders in sign language interpreters. *Journal of Occupational Medicine* 34 (3): 257–264.

Punnett, L., J. M. Robins, D. H. Wegman, and W. M. Keyserling. 1985. Soft-tissue disorders in the upper limbs of female garment workers. *Scandinavian Journal of Work and Environmental Health* 11 (6): 417–425.

Spurgeon, A., J. M. Harrington, and C. L. Cooper. 1997. Health and safety problems associated with long working hours: A review of the current position. *Occupational and Environmental Medicine* 54 (6): 367–375.

Chapter 14: Beating RSI: A Five-Step Protection Plan

Bernacki, E. J., and S. P. Tsai. 1996. Managed care for workers' compensation: Three years of experience in an "employee choice" state. *Journal of Occupational and Environmental Medicine* 38 (11): 1091–1097.

Bernard, B. P., ed. 1997. *Musculoskeletal Disorders and Workplace Factors: A Critical Review of Epidemiologic Evidence for Work-Related Musculoskeletal Disorders of the Neck, Upper Extremity, and Low Back*. Washington, D.C.: U.S. Department of Health and Human Services, Public Health Service, Centers for Disease Control and Prevention, National Institute for Occupational Safety and Health.

Leigh, J. P., S. B. Markowitz, M. Fahs, C. Shin, and P. J. Landrigan. 1997. Occupational injury and illness in the United States: Estimates of costs, morbidity, and mortality. *Archives of Internal Medicine* 157 (14): 1557–1568.

Internet Resources

Typing Injury FAQ

http://www.tifaq.org/organizations
A list of a wide range of governmental and private organizations related to RSI. Includes documents from the technical literature, plus useful advice in nontechnical form. This a good primary source for finding relevant Web sites.

National Coalition on Ergonomics

http://www.ncergo.org
An organization of associations and businesses interested in sound ergonomics.

Office of Ergonomic Research Committee

http://www.oerc.org
An association of companies devoted to research in ergonomics.

Human Factors and Ergonomics Society

http://hfes.org/
An advocacy organization promoting knowledge and exchange of ideas about ergonomics and the use of such knowledge in designing systems to ensure effectiveness, safety, and ease of use.

Coalition of New Office Technology

http://www.ctdrn.org/cnot

An organization focusing on office technology, particularly emphasizing women workers.

Association of Repetitive Motion Syndromes (ARMS)

http://www.certifiedpst.com/arms/

A nonprofit charity that works as a national clearinghouse for support and information to at-risk workers, their employers, workers' compensation professionals, the press, and the public concerning preventive, therapeutic, medical, and legal aspects of repetitive motion syndromes.

Information about Treatment and RSI Educational Materials

http://www.lisasattler.com

CTD Resource Network, Inc.

http://www.ctdrn.org

CTDRN brings together existing, online educational publications and provides a vehicle to more directly assist those suffering from, or at risk of, cumulative trauma disorders.

University of Michigan Rehabilitation Engineering Research Center

http://umrerc.engin.umich.edu/jobdatabase/default.asp

The overall goal of the RERC is to prevent disability associated with musculoskeletal disorders and aging.

General Scientific References on RSI

Further references for those interested in additional scientific research on RSI.

Apfelberg, D. B., and S. J. Larson. 1973. Dynamic anatomy of the ulnar nerve at the elbow. *Journal of Plastic and Reconstructive Surgery* 51: 79–81.

Armstrong T. J. 1983. An ergonomics guide to carpal tunnel syndrome. In *Ergonomics Guides,* ed. T. J. Armstrong. Fairfax, VA: American Industrial Hygiene Association.

Armstrong, T. J., P. Buckle, L. J. Fine, et al. 1993. A conceptual model for work-related neck and upper-limb musculoskeletal disorders. *Scandinavian Journal of Work and Environmental Health* 19: 73–84.

Begg, R. E. 1980. Epicondylitis or tennis elbow. *Orthopaedic Review* 9: 33–42.

Benjamin, M., and J. Ralphs. 1995. Functional and developmental anatomy of tendons and ligaments. In *Repetitive Motion Disorders of the Upper Extremity,* ed. S. L. Gordon, S. J. Blair, L. J. Fine, 185–203. Rosemont, Ill.: American Academy of Orthopedic Surgeons.

Carlson, B. M. 1995. The satellite cell and skeletal muscle regeneration: The degeneration and regeneration cycle in repetitive motion disorders of the upper extremity. American Academy of Orthopedic Surgeons Symposium, Rosemont, Ill. 313–322.

Coonrad, R. W., and W. R. Hooper. 1973. Tennis elbow: Its source, natural history, conservative and surgical management. *Journal of Bone and Joint Surgery* 55A: 1177–1182.

Coote, H. 1861. Exostosis of the left transverse process of the seventh cervical vertebrae, surrounded by blood vessels and nerves, successful removal. *Lancet* 1: 360–361.

Dennett, X., and H. J. Fry. 1988. Overuse syndrome: A muscle biopsy study. *Lancet* 1 (8591): 905–908.

Finkelstein, H. 1930. Stenosing tenovaginitis at the radial styloid process. *Journal of Bone and Joint Surgery* 12: 509.

Fishbein, M., and S. E. Middlestadt, with V. Oltati, et al. 1988. Medical problems among ICSOM musicians: Overview of a national survey. *Medical Problems of Performing Artists* 3: 1–8.

Foletti, G., and F. Regli. 1995. Characteristics of chronic headaches after whiplash injury. *Presse Medicale* 24 (24):1121–1123.

Fridén, J., M. Sjöström, and B. Erblom. 1983. Myofibrillar damage following intense eccentric exercise in man. *International Journal of Sports Medicine* 4: 45–51.

Gilliat, R. W., P. M. LeQuesne, V. Logue, and A. J. Sumner. 1970. Wasting of the hand associated with a cervical rib or band. *Journal of Neurology and Neurosurgical Psychiatry* 33: 615–624.

Goldenberg, D. L. 1992. Controversies in fibromyalgia and myofascial pain syndrome. In *Evaluation and Treatment of Chronic Pain*. 2nd ed. ed. G. M. Arnoff, 165–175. Baltimore: Williams & Wilkins.

Guay, A. H. 1998. Commentary: Ergonomically related disorders in dental practice. *Journal of the American Dental Association* 129 (2): 184–186.

Hochberg, F. H., S. U. Harris, and T. R. Blattert. 1990. Occupational hand cramps: Professional disorders of motor control. *Hand Clinic* 6 (3): 417.

Hochberg, F. H., R. D. Lefert, M. D. Heller, and L. Merriman. 1983. Hand difficulties among musicians. *Journal of the American Medical Association* 249: 1896.

Ireland DCR. Repetition strain injury: the Australian experience–1992 update. *Journal of Hand Surgery* 1995; 20A:S53–S56.

Jordan, S. E., S. S. Ahn, J. A. Freischlag, H. A. Gelabert, and H. I. Machleder. 2000. Selective botulinum chemodenervation of the scalene muscles for treatment of neurogenic thoracic outlet syndrome. *Annals of Vascular Surgery* 14: 365–369.

Juvonen, T., J. Satta, P. Laitala, K. Luukkonen, and J. Nissinen. 1995. Anomalies at the thoracic outlet are frequent in the general population. *American Journal of Surgery* 170: 33–37.

Kelsey, J. L., P. B. Githens, S. D. Walter, W. O. Southwick, U. Neil, T. R.

Holford, A. M. Ostfeld, ct al. 1984. An epidemiological study of acute prolapsed cervical intervertebral disc. *Journal of Bone and Joint Surgery* 66A: 907–914.

Kendall, E. P., B. K. McCreary. 1983. *Muscles: Testing and Function.* Baltimore: Williams & Wilkins.

Kondo, K., C. A. Molgaard, L. T. Kurland, and B. M. Onofrio. 1981. Protruded intervertebral cervical disk: Incidence and affected cervical level in Rochester, Minnesota, 1950 through 1974. *Minnesota Medicine* 64: 751–753.

Lapidus, P. W., and R. Fenton. 1952. Stenosing tenovaginitis at the wrist and fingers: Report of 423 cases in 369 patients with 354 operations. *Archives of Surgery* 64: 475–487.

Larsen, R. D., N. Takagishi, and J. L. Posch. 1960. The pathogenesis of Dupuytren's contracture. *Journal of Bone and Joint Surgery* 42A: 993–1007.

Leach, R. E., and J. K. Miller. 1987. Lateral and medial epicondylitis of the elbow. *Clinical Sports Medicine* 6: 259–272.

Lederman, R. J., and L. H. Calabrese. 1986. Overuse syndromes in instrumentalists. *Medical Problems of Performing Artists* 1: 7.

Linburg, R. M., and B. E. Comstock. 1979. Anomalous tendon slips from the flexor pollicis longus to the flexor digitorum profundus. *Journal of Hand Surgery* 4A: 79–83.

Lister, G. D., R. B. Belsole, and H. E. Kleinert. 1979. The radial tunnel syndrome. *Journal of Hand Surgery* 4: 52–60.

Liu, J. E., A. J. Tahmoush, D. B. Roos, and R. J. Schwartzman. 1995. Shoulder-arm pain from cervical bands and scalene muscle anomalies. *Journal of Neurological Sciences* 128: 175–180.

Machleder, H. I.: 1998. Introduction to neurovascular compression syndromes at the thoracic outlet. In *Vascular Disorders of the Upper Extremity.* 3rd ed., ed. H. I. Machleder, 109–135, Mount Kisco, N.Y.: Futura.

———. 1998. Neurogenic thoracic outlet compression syndrome. In *Vascular Disorders of the Upper Extremity*, 3rd ed., ed. H. I. Machleder, 131–135. Mount Kisco, N.Y.: Futura.

Machleder, H. I., F. Moll, and A. Verity. 1986. The anterior scalene muscle in thoracic outlet compression syndrome: Histochemical and morphometric studies. *Archives of Surgery* 121: 1141–1144.

Mackinnon, S. E., and C. B. Novak. 1994. Clinical commentary: Pathogenesis of cumulative trauma disorder. *Journal of Hand Surgery* 19A (5): 873–883.

————. 1996. Evaluation of the patient with thoracic outlet syndrome. *Seminars in Thoracic and Cardiovascular Surgery* 8 (2): 190–200.

————. 1997. Clinical perspective: Repetitive strain in the workplace. *Journal of Hand Surgery* 22A (1): 2–18.

Maeda, K. 1977. Occupational cervicobrachial disorder and its causative factors. *Journal of Human Ergology* 6: 193–202.

Maeda, K., S. Horiguchi, and M. Hosokawa. 1982. History of the studies on occupational cervicobrachial disorders in Japan and remaining problems. *Journal of Human Ergology* 11: 17–29.

Mannheimer, J. S., and R. M. Rosenthal. 1991. Acute and chronic postural abnormalities as related to craniofacial pain and temporomandibular disorders. *Dental Clinics of North America* 35: 185–208.

Marklin, R. W., and J. F. Monroe. 1998. Quantitative biomechanical analysis of wrist motion in bone-trimming jobs in the meat packing industry. *Ergonomics* 41 (2): 227–237.

Mauro, A. 1961. Satellite cell of skeletal muscle fibers. *Journal of Biophysical and Biochemical Cytology* 9: 493–495.

Moldover, V. 1978. Tinel's sign—its characteristics and significance. *Journal of Bone and Joint Surgery* 60A: 412.

Newmark, J., and F. H. Hochberg. 1987. Isolated painless manual incoordination in 57 musicians. *Journal of Neurology and Neurosurgical Psychiatry* 50: 291.

Pascarelli, E. F. 1998. Evaluation and treatment of repetitive motion disorders. In *Vascular Disorders of the Upper Extremity,* 3rd ed., ed. H. I. Machleder, 171–196. Mount Kisco, N.Y.: Futura.

Pascarelli, E., and J. Kella. 1993. Soft-tissue injuries related to use of the computer keyboard: A clinical study of 53 severely injured persons. *Journal of Occupational Medicine* 35: 5.

Phalen, G. S. 1951. Spontaneous compression of the median nerve at the wrist. *Journal of the American Medical Association* 145: 1128–1133.

————. 1966. The carpal tunnel syndrome. *Journal of Bone and Joint Surgery* 48A: 211–228.

————. 1968. The carpal tunnel syndrome: Seventeen years' experience in diagnosis and treatment of 654 hands. *Journal of Bone and Joint Surgery* 48A: 211–228.

Regan, W. D., and B. F. Morrey. 1994. Entrapment neuropathies about the elbow. In *Orthopaedic Sports Medicine: Principles and Practice,* ed. J. C. DeLee and D. Drez Jr., 1 :844–859. Philadelphia: W. B. Saunders.

Roos, D. B. 1976. Congenital anomalies associated with thoracic outlet syndrome: Anatomy, symptoms, diagnosis, and treatment. *American Journal of Surgery* 132: 771–778.

————. 1979. New concepts of thoracic outlet syndrome that explain etiology, symptoms, diagnosis, and treatment. *Vascular Surgery* 13: 313–321.

————. 1980. Pathophysiology of congenital anomalies in thoracic outlet syndrome. *Acta Chirurgica Belgica* 79: 353–361.

————. 1989. Overview of thoracic outlet syndromes in vascular disorders of the upper extremity. In *Vascular Disorders of the Upper Extremity*, 2nd ed., ed. H. I. Machleder, 155–177. Mount Kisco, NY: Futura.

————. 1989. Thoracic outlet nerve compression. In *Vascular Surgery*, ed. R. B. Rutherford, 858–875. Philadelphia: W. B. Saunders.

Rosenman, K. D., J. C. Gardiner, J. Wang, J. Biddle, A. Hogan, M. J. Reilly, K. Roberts, et al. 2000. Why most workers with occupational repetitive trauma do not file for workers' compensation. *Journal of Occupational and Environmental Medicine* 42 (1): 25–34.

Schwartzman, R. J. 1991. Brachial plexus traction injuries. *Frontiers Hand Rehabilitation* 7: 547–556.

Seddon, J. H. 1943. Three types of nerve injury. *Brain* 66: 237–288.

Sheon, R. P. 1997. Repetitive strain injury. 1. An overview of the problem and the patients. The Goff Group. *Postgraduate Medicine* 102 (4): 53–56:62–68.

Silverstein, B. A., D. S. Stetson, W. M. Keyserling, and L. J. Fine. 1997. Work-related musculoskeletal disorders: Comparison of data sources for surveillance. *American Journal of Industrial Medicine* 31 (5): 600–608.

Simons, D. G. 1988. Myofascial pain syndromes: Where are we? Where are we going? *Archives of Physical Medicine Rehabilitation* 69: 207–212.

Spurling, R. G., and W. R. Scoville. 1944. Lateral rupture of the cervical intervertebral disc. *Surgery Gynecology and Obstetrics* 78: 350–357.

Stone, W. E. 1986. Occupational overuse syndrome in other countries. *Journal of Occupational Health and Safety Aust NZ* 3 (4): 400.

Sucher, B. M. 1990. Thoracic outlet syndrome: A myofascial variant: Part 2. Treatment. *Journal of the American Osteopathic Association* 90: 810–823.

Sucher, B. M., and D. M. Heath. 1993. Thoracic outlet syndrome: A myofascial variant: Part 3. Structural and postural considerations. *Journal of the American Osteopathic Association* 93: 334–345.

Tenner, E. 1996. *Why Things Bite Back: Technology and the Revenge of Unintended Consequences.* New York: Alfred A. Knopf.

Veldman, P. H., H. M. Reynen, I. E. Arntz, R. J. Goris. 1993. Signs and symptoms of reflex sympathetic dystrophy: Prospective study of 829 patients. *Lancet* 342: 1012–1016.

Weigert, B. J., A. A. Rodriguez, R. G. Radwin, and J. Sherman. 1999. Neuromuscular and psychological characteristics in subjects with work-related forearm pain. *American Journal of Physical Medicine and Rehabilitation* 78 (6): 545–551.

Wilshire, W. H. 1860. Supernumerary first rib: Clinical records. *Lancet* 2: 633.

Zohn, D. A. 1988. *Musculoskeletal Pain: Diagnosis and physical treatment,* 2nd ed., 183–188. Boston: Little, Brown.

Zuger, A. 1999. Are doctors losing touch with hands-on medicine? Science Times, *New York Times.* July 13.

Index